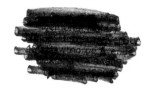
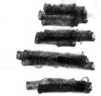

An ~~excellent and fascing~~ look

inside the ICU

Imagine that you (or a family member) have just been thrust into the Intensive Care Unit of the local hospital. You have no idea what to expect or what you need to ask. Why are all the alarms sounding? What are all these computer monitors? How do you navigate this strange world?

Perhaps you are a nurse and have always been intrigued by the real life events of the ICU. This book will help you learn more about what really happens behind those curtains. What does the ICU nurse do in life and death situations?

This book will also captivate those who enjoy reading and watching medical dramas. Share the author's experiences when the tables are turned and she, herself, becomes a patient.

Along with stories and anecdotes about helping her patients, readers will also discover how several patients helped this professional learn a few lessons as well.

D1475076

INSIDE THE ICU

INSIDE THE ICU

A Nursing Perspective

Melody M. Stenrose

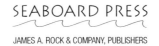

SEABOARD PRESS

JAMES A. ROCK & COMPANY, PUBLISHERS

Inside the ICU: A Nursing Perspective by Melody M. Stenrose

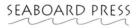

SEABOARD PRESS

is an imprint of JAMES A. ROCK & CO., PUBLISHERS

Inside the ICU: A Nursing Perspective
copyright ©2009 by Melody M. Stenrose

Special contents of this edition copyright ©2009 by Seaboard Press

© Andrei Malov | Dreamstime.com

Address comments and inquiries to:
SEABOARD PRESS
900 South Irby Street, #508
Florence, SC 29501

E-mail:
jrock@rockpublishing.com   lrock@rockpublishing.com
Internet URL: www.rockpublishing.com

Trade Paperback ISBN: 978-1-59663-717-7

Library of Congress Control Number: 2008931155

Printed in the United States of America

First Edition: 2009

This book is dedicated to

my mother-in-law

Marie

also a nurse

ACKNOWLEDGMENTS

First and foremost, to my husband and best friend, Mark, who initiated the idea of sharing my stories with others who could benefit from my experiences. His unlimited support kept me going through the uncertain process.

And to my parents, Johnnie and Ruthmary Hardy, who have always encouraged me to do what made me happy and follow my dreams. I could not have come as far in life as I have without my loving parents.

For the relentless encouragement of my friend and neighbor, Cynthia Katona—English professor and author of several books—who pushed me to move forward with publication when I was doubting myself.

And special thanks to the California Nurses Association, who stood up for me and helped fight for my right to publish the book and tell the world what nurses do on a daily basis.

And finally to all the nurses—not just ICU nurses—for their devotion and dedication to caring for those who cannot care for themselves.

Contents

Introduction

Nursing is a very satisfying career. Nursing in the ICU is a very rewarding yet stressful component of the nursing profession. The intensive care unit is the unit within the hospital where the sickest patients go, those who require a higher level of care. ICU's may be called the intensive care unit, the critical care unit, the coronary care unit, or the cardiac care unit. Some hospitals have several units and separate them into surgical ICUs, medical ICUs, and neuro ICUs. Unlike the other units within the hospital, where nurses care for five or six patients, each nurse in the ICU only cares for one or two because those patients are so critically ill that they consume all of the nurses' undivided time. Sometimes patients in the ICU are so sick and unstable that there are two nurses in the room providing minute-to-minute care for that one critically ill patient.

Often, after working my twelve-hour shift in the ICU, I would come home and share my day with my husband. Sometimes he wouldn't even ask how my day was, but I would still tell him about each of the rewarding and stressful events. I found that retelling what happened at work was like a de-briefing. I could share my thoughts and feelings and I would feel better. The stress and emotions that were often built up during the day could be released at home during this de-briefing time.

One day as I was retelling my experience to my husband, he sat and listened attentively, as usual. When I was finished with the amazing tale of the day, he looked at me, making sure the stress signs were gone from my face and said, "You should write some of this down. You could write a book."

And the seed was planted—a few days later I started thinking of all the different experiences I have lived through while working in the ICU. I sat down and put in writing one of the stories I had recently shared with my husband. From that day on, it all started coming together.

I wrote this book for one reason—to enlighten readers about the inner world of the ICU. By sharing these stories, which chronicle more than twenty-five years working as an ICU nurse, I sincerely hope that all readers will benefit from my experiences. While writing this book, I've kept in mind that these readers will generally fall into two distinct categories: professional health-care workers (mostly nurses) and the general public.

For professionals, my hope is that *all* nurses, not just those with experience in the ICU, will benefit from the lessons I've learned during my career. I also hope that my narrative will "demystify" the activities in the ICU and help the general reader gain a better understanding by detailing what really happens in this unit and what, exactly, an ICU nurse experiences on a day-to-day basis.

Finally, I hope that this book will help initiate some thoughtful conversations concerning medical decisions and painful end-of-life choices, which are sometimes unnecessarily delayed and often not addressed in a timely manner.

Because I've written for both nurses and the average person, this book may sometimes appear a little schizophrenic (a mental disorder that involves illogical thinking and disorganized thoughts). On one page, my thoughts might be directed toward the nurse and then the next page or chapter may be aimed at the layperson. I did this because I feel strongly that both groups can benefit from every chapter in some way.

In this book, when I talk about nurses, I am referring to ICU nurses because the ICU is the basis of this story. When I talk about nurses in other areas, I will either specify the specialty area or refer to the floor nurse. In the hospital, the ICU is the "unit" and the other areas are the "floors"—medical floor, surgical floor, and orthopedic floor.

There are many, many wonderful men who have chosen a career in nursing. I admire all of them. Likewise, there are uncountable great women doctors. But, for the sake of clarity and simplicity, when occasional generic references are made to these professionals, I'll refer to nurses as women and doctors as men.

In this book, I write about my own personal experiences. Each incident has taught me something, or has a special meaning to me. Some of the events are from my early years in nursing and I reflect back at them and contemplate how I could have done better. Now, in my more recent years, because I have grown and learned from my own experiences, I handle each event in hopefully, a better way resulting in positive outcomes.

In this book, I write about real events and real people. All the names and identifying characteristics have been changed in order to maintain confidentiality. Likewise, some of the details have been modified in order to protect the privacy of those involved. Any similarities between any real person and any of the characters in this book are purely coincidental, as many of these events and scenarios happen every day in many hospitals. I have chosen to use real events as the basis for each chapter, because each of these scenarios tells a different story, and each can provide a meaningful experience for the reader, just as they were for me. I hope that each and every chapter will provide you, the reader, with an insight into what the ICU nurse does on a day-to-day basis, and an insight into the real life—*Inside The ICU*.

CHAPTER 1

In the Beginning

*My personal journey toward becoming a nurse and
entering into the rewarding field of ICU nursing.*

Whenever I'm asked how old I was when I decided to become a nurse. I always respond, "I don't know." Honestly, I really cannot identify when I made that decision. My first memories were when I was about eight-years-old. My best friend, who lived next door, was diabetic. I was intrigued when she administered her insulin shots. I would watch as she checked her urine for sugar, with those little fizzy tabs. I was always interested in everything related to her disease and the special needs she required. That may have been the beginning of my quest to be a nurse.

I think I was born to be a nurse. I feel strongly that good nurses are born, not made. You cannot teach someone to be a compassionate nurse. Some people are destined to be teachers, while others are naturally good engineers, but nurses are naturally evolved from an early desire to help others. Many, like myself, are naturally destined to be nurses, from an early age. To be a good nurse, one must have a certain caring personality and a helping nature. You must be able to *give* of yourself, before *thinking* of yourself.

Good nurses do not enter this profession because they can make money, or because they can work part time, or because they can work variable shifts. In fact, working variable shifts, weekends, and holidays are one of the disadvantages of the nursing profession. For those of us who are in this profession because of the innate love of nursing, the evenings, weekends, and holidays are just one of the things we have to endure in order to do what we love doing.

Nursing is not a profession that one can pick out of a college catalog. It is a chosen profession based on a desire or a yearning. Nursing is a hard, labor-intensive job that requires a lot of tasks that are not appealing to many people. In fact, many of the tasks are not appealing to those of us who do them on a daily basis, but we do them because we love the job. Those who enter the field of nursing for reasons other than for caring for others, are in this profession for the wrong reason. Those are the nurses who may not be happy, and who might not provide the quality care that is expected and deserved.

A good nurse must possess a tender, patient personality. Nursing requires hard work, undesirable tasks, and daily frustration, because you may not always be able to provide the best care you know you can give. Most of all, nursing requires compassion and giving. A good nurse is in the profession just for the personal gratification that comes at the end of the day, when you look back and see that you've made a difference.

My Beginning

Since I had decided to become a nurse at an early age, I started taking high school courses that would prepare me for college. As I started my college prep courses in high school, I also started my quest to become a volunteer at the local hospital. I was disappointed to learn that I had to wait until I was sixteen. A few days after my sixteenth birthday, I was at the local hospital filling out the needed application. I was almost as eager to sign up to be a hospital volunteer as I was to get my driver's license. I became a "Blue Miss" and started helping at the front desk and in the gift shop at the hospital. This was as close as I could get to the patients at that time. I continued my volunteer work throughout my high school years.

My senior year of high school brought me one step closer to my goal. I took an occupational training course that taught the basics of how to be a Certified Nursing Assistant. To be a nursing assistant was yet another stepping-stone toward becoming a nurse. Taking vital signs, giving baths, turning and ambulating patients were skills I learned in order to obtain my nursing assistant certificate. When I acquired my first job as a nurse's aide in a local nursing home, I felt confident that I was on my way to a career in nursing. Working as a nurse's aide just reinforced my love of nursing. It didn't matter that those debilitated old folks couldn't talk to me and perhaps didn't even know that I was there. It didn't matter that no one came to visit those bed-ridden, emaciated skeletons with bedsores. It didn't matter that these elderly human beings could no longer provide a productive contribution to society. What did matter was that I was turning, feeding and bathing these helpless people, and that I was providing them with what they could not provide for themselves. What did matter was that the others, those who did know that I was there, were appreciative that I was dressing them and assisting them to their wheel chairs so they could go to the community room for meals and activities. It mattered that I was helping those who still could participate, could enjoy the company of the other residents, and converse and play bingo. I enjoyed this first step of my nursing career. I was helping these people who could not help themselves.

As I was finishing my senior year of high school, I applied at the local junior college for admission to the nursing program. I completed the application, the letters of recommendations, and survived the personal interviews. I was ecstatic to learn that I was one of forty individuals, from a pool of over one-hundred and fifty who were accepted to the nursing program.

Three years later, at the age of twenty-one, I had graduated, passed my state boards, and was on my way to being a real nurse. I landed my first job, with an interim permit, in a new-graduate program. New-graduate programs are set up for nurses directly out of school. Unlike orientation programs for experienced nurses, which provide one to two weeks of orientation, these programs provide a six to eight week extended amount of time with an on-unit preceptor for the new nurse. I worked closely for six weeks with an experienced nurse, who helped me learn what was not possible to learn in school: the prioritizing, the organizing, the caring, and most of all personal touches needed to be a good nurse. *Patty, thank you for the beginning you gave me.*

After a year working evenings and nights as a "float" nurse—one who works on a different unit each day—I applied for a full-time day shift position on a medical floor. That medical unit was being converted to a telemetry unit and included the installation of cardiac monitors and the extensive education of the nursing staff. During my interview for this new position, the manager asked me what my career plans were. I remember telling her that in about ten years, I hoped to move into ICU—but not for at least ten years. After all, I had only been a nurse for a year; those ICU patients were still scary to me.

When I got that job, I was required to take classes to learn how to interpret telemetry rhythms. That was a big deal back then, early in my career. Now, only one year into my career, I was not only a nurse, but was also specializing as a telemetry nurse. I would be taking care of patients who had cardiac monitors and I would be responsible for interpreting the rhythms. Today, telemetry is a common occurrence and not as big of a deal as it was then. Currently, many hospitals have telemetry on every unit and many newly graduated nurses are required to learn telemetry right out of school.

I worked on that telemetry floor for another couple of years, when one day I came to work and was told that I was to float into the ICU. Nurses generally do not like to float from one unit to another. Most nurses are hired to work on a specific floor and/or unit. Many units specialize in one area such as medical, surgical, orthopedic, oncology and so on. However, when one unit has fewer patients than another, the unit with fewer patients must send a nurse to the unit that has more. This is called floating. In my case, since I at least knew telemetry, the nursing supervisor decided I was the best choice to send into the ICU.

I don't remember much of that first day in ICU. I'm sure they assigned me to the least critical patients, and I'm sure the charge nurse had her eye on me every minute. Today, no one gets floated to ICU without some orientation. The nurse is oriented to the unit and assigned a resource nurse to assist her with any tasks she may not be comfortable performing. The resource nurse also assures the float nurse is competent to perform the skills and has the abilities required to care for patients in this higher level area. What I do remember about my first experience in ICU was what actually happened the next day. When I came back to work the following morning, I was told to go back to ICU again. I didn't like that idea; I was not comfortable in that unit. I called the nursing supervisor, who made the staffing decisions, and pleaded with her not to send me back to that unit. I suggested that she send anyone else but me, and she did. I went back to my telemetry unit, where I was comfortable, and some other poor soul had to go to that scary place called ICU.

Two years later, I was floating into ICU on a regular basis. So regularly, that when a full time position became available, I applied and was granted the position. Within four years of graduating, I was an ICU nurse. I have worked in ICU ever since and now would not want to work anywhere else. Now when floated out of ICU, I complain for similar reasons. I am not comfortable in that unit, any unit but ICU.

The ICU Nurse

ICU nurses are different from other nurses, but what makes the ICU nurse different? Is it that she deals day after day with patients who are on the brink of death? Is it that she deals daily with grieving family members who are about to lose their loved ones? Is it that she deals with patients on a daily basis who, fifty years ago, would not have survived their illnesses? Is it that she must often act instinctively and immediately in order to prevent death? I'm not sure what makes the ICU nurse different, but I am sure she is

Because of the more demanding level of care required, the ICU nurse is expected to deal with critical situations on a daily basis. Because of the intensive nature of the job, the ICU nurse is required to have a higher level of expertise and critical thinking skills. As a result of this higher level of expertise, other nurses throughout the hospital look to the ICU nurses for assistance and clinical support. Often, a floor nurse will call the ICU nurse and consult regarding a patient who has developed difficulty breathing or who has just had an irregular heart rhythm. Problem situations, deteriorating conditions, changes in status, may all initiate consultation with the ICU nurse from other nurses.

Not only do the other nurses depend on the ICU nurse for clinical support, so do the doctors. Most doctors spend fifteen to twenty minutes with the patient each day; the nurse spends eight to twelve hours with that same patient. The doctor depends on the assessment skills, the critical thinking, and the educated opinions of the nurse to help provide the best care for his patients. Situations occur on a daily basis that require the nurse to make snap decisions in order to save lives. Because sometimes events change drastically and suddenly, the nurse may not have time to consult with the physician. She must depend on her own knowledge, her own skills, and her own gut feelings to guide her rather than the physician. Immediate actions are frequently needed to save the life of the patient for which she is responsible. This, perhaps, is what makes the ICU nurse a different breed of nurse. Because we deal with life-and-death situations daily, because we take care of the sickest patients, because other nurses look to us for clinical support and so many others depend on us, some may think we are a step above.

The ICU nurse is not a step above; she is simply a different kind of nurse and usually a different type of person. It takes a special person to be a nurse, and each nurse has to find her niche in nursing. There are many kinds of nurses because there are many *areas* of nursing: operating room, labor & delivery, emergency, oncology, med/surg, burn units, and so forth. Each area requires a special person, a special nurse. The ICU is simply a unique area and requires an exceptional type of nurse.

ICU nursing is a world of its own. Just as I was afraid, twenty-five years ago, when I was first sent to the ICU, I find many "young" nurses are also afraid of "my" ICU today. Because the patients in ICU are sicker and more unstable than any other patients in the hospital, it is an intimidating place, not only for inexperienced nurses, but for families and patients as well. The new ICU nurse comes into the unit, eager to learn, eager to grow, and eager to develop new skills. After attending several classes, these new ICU nurses go through an extensive orientation period that will help them obtain the skills and knowledge needed to perform this higher level of care. Most new ICU nurses have worked on a medical or surgical floor prior to entering ICU. This has afforded them the experience they'll need to provide basic nursing care. In the ICU, they are stepping up to a new level of expectation in nursing.

ICU nurses must have diligent critical thinking skills. Critical thinking is the ability to examine a situation and pull all the pieces of the puzzle together. Too often, nurses will look at a patient, see what is wrong, but are unable to determine the cause of the situation or identify what needs to be done. Critical thinking requires that the ICU nurse quickly identify the problem, the source of the problem as well as the solution. Critical thinking requires that the nurse consider all aspects of what *has* happened, what has *not* happened, and what *needs* to happen in order to provide quality care for her patient.

For example, nurses monitor patient's vital signs. When the blood pressure drops, some nurses will call and inform the doctor without considering all of the reasons. The nurse who uses good critical thinking skills will monitor vital signs and when the blood pressure drops, she will call the doctor, inform him of the patients low blood pressure and provide him with the possible reasons for the change. And, she will also provide solutions that might help solve the problem in the future. This is the difference between a nurse who simply provides care, and one who provides care based on critical thinking skills.

Critical thinking and assertiveness are important skills for the ICU nurse because she cares for patients whose condition can change very quickly at any time. Doctors make rounds daily and sometimes twice a day in ICU. The doctor assesses the patient, reviews the daily labs and test results, consults with the nurse, and makes a plan for the day. Then the doctor writes the orders for what the nurse will do for the patient. These orders will include tests and medications and any nursing interventions that will be done in his absence, so when he comes back, hopefully the patient's condition has improved.

Frequently things do not go the way the doctor would like. The patient's condition changes and the nurse must call to inform him of the changes. She must communicate the assessment, the vital signs, the complaints, the symptoms, and the test results, to the doctor. She must tell him what she is observing, what is wrong with the patient, and what she thinks is happening. And sometimes she must offer suggestions to elicit the appropriate interventions over the phone. The nurse must interrupt the doctor during his other activities, sometimes sleep, and tell him "This is what I see, this is what I think, and this is what we need to do." At times, the doctor does not provide orders for what the nurse knows is best for the patient. At these times, she will elicit support from more experienced physicians or the medical directors, in order to assure the patient is receiving what is needed. The nurse must sometimes, for the benefit of the patient, go up the chain of command; seek additional support to assure the patient is getting what is necessary to survive.

Years ago, when I was a new ICU nurse, I remember my mother coming home from her doctor's appointment. She told me that she had shared with her family practitioner that I was working in the ICU. He told her that ICU nurses are the greatest. "If you ever want to know what's happening with your patient, you ask the ICU nurse. Those girls know what they're doing." Now over twenty-five years later, I know exactly what he meant.

What exactly does the ICU nurse do that makes her different? She takes the extra step. When a patient is in acute respiratory distress, some nurses might call the doctor, get orders for labs or x-rays, then initiate the orders. The ICU nurse will call for the lab test and while waiting for the results of the tests, she will rally the troops to be ready to perform the intervention she is anticipating the doctor will order. As soon as she phones the doctor with the lab results, everyone is positioned and ready to initiate the treatments that she has already anticipated will be ordered by the physician. If a patient goes into a life-threatening arrhythmia, some nurses might call a Code Blue, initiate CPR and wait for the code team to arrive. The ICU nurse will call a Code Blue, take charge of the situation by commanding the first person who walks into the room to start CPR, while she shocks the patient and administers the first medication before the code team has a chance to arrive. The ICU nurse must think rapidly and intervene even more rapidly. That is why we, ICU nurses, are different. The community puts doctors on a pedestal, and often it seems that the ICU nurses are holding the doctors up there on those pedestals.

CHAPTER 2

Tour the ICU— Don't Let It Be Scary

A brief explanation of what to expect in the ICU can alleviate some of the fright.

The intensive care unit is a familiar place to those of us who work there day after day. But for many, the intensive care unit may be alarming. When you go to any new area—someplace you've never been before—you enter with caution. As you enter the ICU, you may see things you have never witnessed. Whether you're a nurse entering the ICU for the first time, or a visitor coming to see a friend or loved one, the ICU can be overwhelming. As a visitor you may be required to travel through what appears to be chaos before you reach your destination. Not only are you uncertain of your surroundings, but also you are anxious because your family member is critically ill.

The nurses become very familiar with the surroundings. We often forget that others who enter our unit are overwhelmed with what they see and what they hear. My own husband won't even come to bring my lunch. He is so uncomfortable with the entire setup that he makes me come out to the car to pick up any items he must deliver. My own husband hears all the recaps of events that I live through on a daily basis. You would think that he would be less distressed because he is familiar with the setting. Even with his familiarity, he still says, "I'm not going in that place."

Whoever said, "Ignorance is bliss" must not have had an opportunity to visit an ICU. "Knowledge is power" when it comes to relieving the stress of our infrequent visitors. If visitors understand the complexity of the activities in the unit—the machinery, the clamor of strange sounds and the duties of each nurse—it may help alleviate some of their anxiety. I hope the information in this chapter will alleviate some of the stress of the first time patients and visitors.

* * *

All patients, when admitted to the ICU, are connected to a variety of monitoring devices. Every patient will have an intravenous catheter (IV), will be attached to an EKG monitor and a blood pressure cuff, and will have their oxygen saturation monitored. The IV catheter is inserted upon admission to the ICU in order to allow us to give fluids and medication directly into the blood stream. Even if the patient does not need IV fluids, we attach a short tubing called a saline lock. This allows quick access just in case the patient should need emergency medications.

The EKG monitor is attached to the chest with five sticky pads. The wires—attached to the bedside monitor—allow the nurse to see the patient's heart rate and cardiac rhythm. The heart rate may be one of the first signs of distress. It goes up when the patient is in pain, has a fever, is anxious, and many more reasons. The cardiac rhythm can indicate cardiac problems, electrolyte imbalance, or other warning signs of trouble. The EKG rhythm is displayed on the monitor at the bedside, and also on the monitor in the centrally located nursing station. Vital signs are monitored more frequently in the ICU than in other areas of the hospital. Blood pressure cuffs often stay on the arm between readings.

Oxygen therapy is also initiated on most ICU patients. To assure an adequate oxygen level, the oxygen saturation (O2 sat) is monitored on a continuous basis. The O2 sat monitor looks like a white band-aid on the finger. This band-aid is attached to a wire that leads to the bedside monitor. A red light shines from the band-aid device, through the finger, toe, or earlobe that it is attached to, and reads the amount of oxygen circulating in the red blood cells of the body. This provides a reading of the concentration of oxygen in the blood, and thus represents the oxygen level within the body.

Every patient in the ICU has a minimum of these four monitoring devices. So every patient has four unfamiliar cords or wires attached to them as soon as they arrive. As you can imagine, these connections make it difficult to maneuver around in bed, or in and out of bed.

In addition to these basic monitoring devices, there are several other ways to monitor patients. We refer to these as "lines." A "line" is usually a tube, an IV, or a monitoring device that is attached to the patient. Each patient may have several lines used to monitor or support in different ways. An arterial line, (art-line) is like an IV, but instead of being placed in a vein, it is inserted into an artery. This is usually in the wrist, but sometimes in another location. The art-line allows us to monitor arterial blood pressure on a minute-to-minute basis. The art-line also provides a convenient access to draw blood without repeatedly sticking the patient over and over.

Central venous pressure lines (CVP line) are also similar to IV's. But, these IV's are inserted in a large central vein, usually in the neck or upper chest. These allow us to administer large volumes of fluids, monitor central venous pressure or fluid balance, and give specialized medications.

Pulmonary artery lines (PA line) are inserted like the CVP line, through a large vein. This line is not a short tubing, but a wire-like device that is threaded through the right side of the heart into the pulmonary artery of the lungs. This important catheter relays pressure readings from the heart and lungs that allow us to monitor fluid balance and the function of the heart. All of these lines are attached to the bedside monitor, displayed on the screen in different colors, and provide the medical team with vital information in order to care for the ICU patient.

Machines are also common around the ICU bed. The most prominent is the monitor that usually hangs on the wall and displays the EKG rhythm, vital signs, and all the pressures and waveforms from the previously mentioned lines. IV pumps will also be at every bedside. IV pumps control the rate of infusions of the fluids and medications (IV drips) that require frequent adjustments and close monitoring to achieve the desired effects. These pumps are important in controlling the rate of infusions for all IV's and medications.

Other machines may or may not be at each bedside. Ventilators are large machines that sit next to the bed and are attached to the patient who requires ventilation support. Ventilators breathe for the patients when they can't breath for themself. Bi-level Positive Airway Pressure machines (Bi-pap) are also ventilator assistant machines but these are smaller and usually on carts. Bi-pap provides less invasive breathing assistance for the patient.

Other machines may be seen around the bedside in ICU. Sequential compression devices are machines that inflate and deflate a leg wrapping to stimulate circulation in the legs. Cooling/warming blankets surge cold or hot water through the mattress to cool or warm the patient. Intracranial pressure (ICP) monitors report the pressure from inside the brain. Intra-aortic balloon pumps and ventricular assist devices are machines that help the heart. There are many machines that sometimes crowd the ICU rooms in order to monitor and provide life support to the patient. Many of these machines and their uses will be explained in this book.

Most distressing about these machines, to most ICU novices, are the alarms. There are many different alarms. All the machines have alarms that will alert the staff when attention is necessary. Each alarm has a different sound and tone. Sometimes family members will sit at the bedside, and each and every time an alarm rings, they will jump up and call for the nurse. They worry that the needs of their family is not being met. They worry that the nurses are not responding to the emergency needs of each and every alarm. But, the nurse knows the reason for all of these alarms, and she knows which ones require immediate attention and which ones can be addressed with less urgency. Even if the nurse is not running to the bedside, she is aware of the reason for each of these unwanted noises. Just as she prioritizes her duties, she will prioritize her response to alarms. She will respond based on the sound of the alert and the importance of the alarm.

For example, the ventilator alarm rings when the patient is coughing, causing an increase in pressure. This will be registered in the nurses mind, and she will most often, wait to see if it resolves. But, when a louder, more high-pitched alarm rings, alerting the nurse that the patient has become disconnected, she will respond immediately. This disconnect alarm will receive a quicker response than the high-pressure alert.

Likewise, the EKG monitor has a variety of alarms. A quiet alert "beep—beep—beep" may advise the nurse that the blood pressure is above or below the set limits. A louder "bong—bong—bong" may be what alerts the nurse that the heart rate is too fast or too slow. And finally, a loud blaring "BONGBONGBONG" notifies all staff of an immediate emergency. These red alarms are attended to immediately, if not at the bedside, at the nurses' station. Most intensive care units have monitoring at the bedside, and also at the centrally located nurses station. Although it appears that no one is aware of the alarms, nurses are acutely tuned to each and every sound and respond accordingly.

The purring of the machines and the buzzing of the alarms cause an unusually high noise level in the ICU. While these mechanical noises are not avoidable, some others are. Staff members conversing with visitors, visitors talking to visitors, and nurses consulting with physicians can also result in an unintentional increase noise level.

Unnecessary sounds and disruptions can be alarming to patients and visiting family members. Awareness of the noise level is the best tool to reduce it. Thus, we should all be aware of the noise level of our conversations in the ICU.

Visitors may also create stress within the ICU. Because patients are more critically ill, visitations may be limited. Immediate family only, for a few minutes at a time, is often the visiting rule. Limiting visits to a few minutes at a time, allows the nurse to provide frequent monitoring and care for the patient. A few minutes at a time allows the patient to rest in between visitors. Family support is important for the sick, but too many family interruptions may hinder the ability of the patient to receive care and rest that is also needed to recuperate. Most patients need their rest more than they need great Uncle John or Cousin Beverly to come and tell them how their day was.

Visiting may be limited because of the needs of the patient, or the needs of nurse to provide care, or the needs of the entire unit. During an emergency, visitors will be restricted in order to provide privacy, or to avoid additional confusion and chaos in the surrounding areas.

The ICU often may appear chaotic, with many things going on at once. Each nurse is caring for her patients who have multiple lines and machines attached. The nurse is either at the bedside providing care, or near the nurses' station monitoring from a distance. Every patient is being monitored and watched at all times.

ICU can be a disturbing place if you don't understand what's happening and what all the tubes and machines are for. Mostly, remember that the nurse will attend to the most urgent issues first. If there is an alarm to attend to, the nurse will address it in the time required based on its urgency. If the nurse is tending to another patient, and an urgent alarm sounds, she will stop what she is doing to address the emergency. If the alarm is a low level alert, she most likely will finish her task before attending to the alert. Rest assured, every nurse is aware of every patient, at every moment. The duty of the family and the visitors are to support the patient, while the nurse provides care. Hopefully a little knowledge and understanding will alleviate some of the stress that is inevitable the first time you visit the ICU.

CHAPTER 3

No Talking Back

*What happens when the patient cannot talk or
communicate with the nurses?*

Communicating is one of our most vital necessities. If we take
that away from our patients, they will have no way to tell us what
they need, no way to tell us what is wrong. Many things that we do
interfere with the ability of our patients to communicate. Surgical
interventions, medications, physical restraints all hamper communication. Many of us avoid communicating with our patients, maybe
because we don't know how, or maybe because we are afraid, or
maybe because we simply don't want to take the time. We are in this
profession, to provide for the sick what they cannot provide for
themselves. If we don't allow these helpless people to communicate
their needs, we put them in danger. We leave them at our mercy to
provide what we think they need, maybe not what they actually
need. Is that fair?

* * *

One of my first patients in ICU was a gentleman named Charles.
Charles was 42-years-old. He was in our ICU for almost two months,
suffering from Guillain-Barré syndrome. Guillian-Barré is an unfortunate affliction that causes an inflammation of the nerves. The
nerves are what carry the messages to and from the brain. How does

17

our brain tell our hand to move? The signals are carried by the nerves to the muscles. If the nerves are not doing their job, the message does not get through to make the muscle contract.

Guillian-Barré sometimes follows a viral infection. A few weeks following the viral infection, the patient develops weakness—minor generalized weakness followed by more significant weakness, and finally, if untreated, total paralysis. The paralysis usually starts with the lower extremities and progresses upward to include the arms and the chest. By the time the effects reach the upper part of the body, the patient has had time to prepare for the possibility of total, yet temporary, paralysis.

Today, modern treatment often prevents Guillian-Barré from progressing to this state of total paralysis. Unfortunately for Charles, he did not wait until the twenty-first century to acquire this atrocious disease.

Charles was transferred into the ICU from the medical floor. His muscle weakness was progressing to the point where his physician wanted him monitored more closely than the nurses could do on the medical floor. Initially, Charles was a very lighthearted guy. As he was wheeled into the ICU, he was joking with the orderly about coming back later to sneak him out of what looked like a dungeon.

I had often thought of the ICU as a dungeon, but this was the first time one of our patients picked up on it as he was entering into our domain. Our ICU is not a very pleasant place to be. The outside walls are tall and full of equipment and electrical outlets. The windows are small, short and wide, positioned strategically along the highest point of the exterior wall. Those inconspicuous windows allow only small bits of daylight through the outdated vertical blinds. Because of the limited natural light, large bright fluorescent lights are the only clue as to whether it is day or night in this tomb of the unknown time. Small, isolated cubicles—not rooms with walls, but simply spaces separated by privacy curtains—line the exterior walls that support those concealed windows.

The nurses' station is positioned along the opposite side of the long narrow unit—secluded by cloudy glass on top of a long counter where frequently needed supplies are stored. None of this design was meant to serve as a peaceful refuge, but rather as a functional shelter.

It didn't take long for all of the nurses to get to know Charles who was a high-powered executive, and was used to calling the shots. He was a tall, well-built, handsome gentleman, who was in control of his life, his job, his family, and up until now, his health. Early in his stay, he would joke about anticipating the role reversal that I was trying to prepare him for. He would tell his wife, "I'm going to be the helpless one, and you will have to take care of me for a change." She was there for him on a daily basis, undivided support, spending all her available time at his bedside.

As the days went by, we monitored the degeneration of Charles' strength. We monitored the deterioration of his lower extremities and compared them to his uppers. We watched the uncoordinated movements of his legs progress to total paralysis, while the fine movements of his arms developed to only gross uncoordinated motions. Each day, we watched him follow the slippery slope into total paralysis. We worked hard to keep his strength up as well as his spirits. All the time we were working and preparing, we were hoping that the progression would stop. No amount of preparation can prepare anyone for total paralysis and the dependence that will develop. No one really knows why Guillian-Barré progresses to total paralysis for some, but stops with limited effects on others. All I could do was wait, as Charles became one of the more unfortunate victims of the disease.

We monitored his pulmonary functions frequently. Watching closely, we could see how his deep breathing progressed to shallow breathing and his lack of deep breaths started causing a build-up of carbon dioxide in his system. As the carbon dioxide built up, Charles became more and more lethargic. For Charles, despite the hard work we did to maintain his chest muscle strength, his condition deterio-

rated. It didn't seem very long before Charles required elective intubation, insertion of a breathing tube that would prevent him from
having a respiratory arrest.

✳ ✳ ✳

Respiratory arrest occurs with the cessation of respirations; that
is, the patient stops breathing. Without breathing, the body will
not function; the organs will starve for the oxygen they need, the
muscles will not contract without oxygen, and cells will gasp for the
nourishment needed to function. Life will cease to exist. To stop
breathing will result in death. What if we are not ready to die, what
if the respiratory arrest is due to an unfortunate accident or illness
resulting in premature death. What then?

When a patient stops breathing, medical personnel rapidly move
into action. Mouth to mouth ventilation—when a living person
places his mouth over the mouth of the lifeless body and breaths air
into the still lungs—is initiated. This life-saving act is performed
without the need of any extra equipment. Risks of disease transmis-
sion must be considered. Mouth-to-mouth resuscitation is not a
favorite way to save a life. For anyone in the medical profession who
has done it—once is enough. It only takes one time to convince
most of us, that this is one act of mercy that we don't ever want to
provide for a stranger again. It's not a task that many want to do,
but we will, if necessary.

Luckily, modern technology provides masks to be used rather than
one's own mouth. The mask is attached to a collapsible bag—an ambu
bag. This mask is placed on the victim's mouth and as the bag is
squeezed, air is pushed into the lungs. This allows for cleaner artificial
ventilation. Whoever invented these masks, deserves to be rewarded.

The most efficient means for ventilation is intubation—the insertion of an endotracheal tube. This tube can be placed into the
mouth of a lifeless body, passed through the vocal cords, into the
trachea or airway. Oxygen can be forced through the endotracheal
tube, commonly call the ET tube. Once the airway is established,
breathing assistance can be more easily achieved.

Ventilators are machines that blow oxygen into the lungs when the patient is not able to perform this basic need. Ventilators provide life to lifeless folks while patiently waiting for the medical personnel to do what they train hard to do—save lives.

Ventilators are a common element in the ICU. Many critically ill patients require ventilator support. Surgical patients may require ventilator support after surgery when unforeseen complications prevent them from coming off the machines in the operating room. Trauma or accidents that result in sudden respiratory arrest require ventilator support. And finally, medical patients may need ventilator support as a bridge to recovery when suffering from illness with chronic lung disease or muscle-weakening diseases.

To the ICU nurses and doctors, intubation is a daily occurrence. The ET tube is inserted into the airway, attached to the ventilator, and the patient is provided with the breathing help needed. Ideally, ventilators are used to bridge the time needed to support the patient through an acute illness. Ideally, patients are on a ventilator for only a few days or maybe a week because long-term ventilator support presents additional problems. These problems can include infection, immobility, weakening of muscles and an increase in risks for other complications.

The ET tube will usually remain in the trachea for less than two weeks. Once this time limit has exceeded, the doctor must consider a more permanent means of airway management for long-term ventilator support. The tracheostomy is the surgical procedure physicians perform to place the breathing tube directly into the neck, rather than threading it through the mouth or nose. The surgeon makes a small incision between the collarbones and inserts a shortened tube directly into the airway. This tube is then attached to the ventilator and the ET tube can be removed from the mouth.

The use of an ET tube or a trach always results in loss of voice. In order to talk, air must pass through the vocal cords in the throat. The movements of these cords create the vibration needed to create sounds. When the air is directed either through the ET tube, bypassing the vocal cords, or enters the airway below the vocal cords through a trach, the contact with the cords is eliminated and the ability to make noise, such as words, is no longer possible—silence is the result.

Talking, verbalizing, expressing, pronouncing, communicating, any way we think of speaking, it's often taken for granted by many of us. Talking is the most basic way of expressing our needs. Calling out, asking for what we need, is one of our basic acts of self-preservation. But what happens when we lose this basic ability? To be without the simplest way to communicate must create an exorbitant degree of stress. Imagine lying in a bed, unable to talk, yell, scream, and unable to move physically. Verbal communication is not possible and *now* you are unable to use your hands to push the button to call the nurse.

* * *

Charles was intubated through his mouth and eventually, because of the longevity of his illness, he earned himself a tracheostomy. Both resulted in his inability to communicate. Because of the time I had to bond with Charles prior to the intubation, I developed an over-protective relationship with him. In the beginning of this difficult time, I would peek in on him every time I would walk by his room, probably more often than necessary, to make sure his desires were addressed. I would stop by on my way home, to make sure he didn't need anything before I left. I would make frequent stops, coming and going, just to say hello.

I felt sorry for Charles. The role that had now been forced upon him was not his choice. He did not ask for this debilitating syndrome that threw him into a helpless state. He did not want to lie in bed, defenseless, nor did he enjoy having a stranger turn, feed, bathe, brush, shave and clean areas of his body that most people don't share. My unhealthy doting quickly transformed Charles into, what I now see, was an overly dependent patient.

Charles lay in bed, day after day, as still as a rug, any signs of movements were gone. Not only had he lost any possibility of physical movement, he had also lost his ability to communicate. His only means of communication was the limited facial movement he had remaining. He used his eyebrows to answer questions. Raising the brows, with wide eyes, alerted me to a positive response. A frown with the brows aggressively joining in the middle would signify his negative reply. His eyes, which were now his only means of communicating, would help proclaim his wants and needs. Those limited expressions worked for a while, but after the challenges of Charles' care were gone and he became just another patient in our unit, I started entering his room less and less often, only going in when I needed to perform some necessary tasks. Now Charles was only receiving attention when I chose to go into his room. Without the ability to call, the previously independent executive was not only dependent on me to provide all of his bodily needs, but he also had to have his needs met when it was convenient for me.

It seemed that his isolation became more of a problem than his lack of communication. He thrived on the constant attention. He yearned for the moment-by-moment interventions. He grieved in loneliness when his wife was not constantly with him. In loneliness, he grasped for the attention of the nurses at all times.

Charles soon realized he needed a way to call; he needed a way to get my attention. He was helpless; his lifeless limbs were useless. No movement was possible, no call bell was available, and no matter how hard he tried, he could not get his eyebrows to call out. Those eyes just would not make the noise he needed them to make to get my withering attention.

Lying there, grieving the loss of attention, Charles soon realized that his eyebrows were not the only facial features that worked. His lips could slightly separate and his tongue still moved. Now that the ET tube had been removed from his mouth, he could move his tongue gently once again. He started making a snapping sound, tapping his tongue against the back of his teeth. This tongue snapping was his new way of communicating. He would snap his tongue as if he was snapping his fingers. He found a new way to get attention, to make a noise, and he could now command a response.

Initially this newfound alert system was a good thing for both of us. I could go about my work as needed, and he could call when he wanted something. This tongue snapping soon became Charles' way of controlling his life once again. He was quickly moving back into the high-powered person he once was. However, I had turned Charles into an overly-dependent person and his dependency was now interfering with my duties as I tried to provide care for other patients in the ICU.

The demanding nature of this dependent patient became an annoyance. I stopped entering his room as often as I had previously. And I stopped doting over his every whim. I moved on, but unfortunately, Charles was not able to move anywhere. I made him into what he was, but now I was unable to follow through with what I had cultivated. I started setting limits. I would do what I had to do, give him a specific time that I would be back and hope that he wouldn't bother me. But, it seemed like every time he saw me walk by his room, he started "snapping." I would make sure he had every thing I thought he needed when I was in the room, but within five minutes that tongue was clicking once again.

I did continue to provide good care for Charles. I made sure he had all his needs met, and I absolutely did not neglect him. But I soon started resenting his ability to communicate. I realized I was more comfortable doing for Charles *what* I wanted to do, *when* I wanted to do it; and not when he wanted me to do things for him. His snapping was becoming more and more annoying. His tongue clicking was out of control. I hated the fact that he was now controlling me. That is why I am an ICU nurse, because I like to be in control. ICU patients require total care and *I* can control that total care.

All that time I had spent preparing Charles for this devastating period was paying off now. He was maintaining his soul and was not falling into a depression as some do. But, he was driving me crazy. I didn't realize I was giving up my control by allowing him to maintain his.

Unfortunately, I quickly learned how to regain that control. Remember, that's why I'm an ICU nurse; I like to have that control.

I decided that I would be the one to control me, Charles couldn't. I still had the physical ability to move, he didn't. I could walk away, he couldn't. I could conveniently be out of earshot when Charles would snap that tongue. I could look the other way as if I didn't hear him. I could stand out of his visual field so he didn't know I was hearing him. I wouldn't need to jump when he called, and I could regain control.

I stopped doting over Charles, started to ignore him and eventually he stopped calling every five minutes. I felt I was weaning him from the overly dependent person he had become. I felt I was doing what was right for him. Eventually, we seemed to come to a happy medium. I continued to care for him, despite this annoying tongue snapping, and he stopped bugging me continuously. His needs were met, in what I considered was a timely manner, and I didn't have to jump so often.

His frame of mind changed during this period of his illness. I could see that he was not as vivacious as he was in the beginning, but I felt he was finally adjusting to his situation. After we came to what I considered an agreeable compromise in our schedule, he slept more; he watched TV instead of paying attention to all of the nursing activities, and he stopped asking for the "little things" that he used to enjoy. Maybe Charles had adjusted to his situation, or maybe he had just given up. Maybe he stopped asking for the little things because I had stopped offering them; but actually, I had stopped paying attention to him. I never stopped attending to his physical needs, but I unknowingly stopped attending to his psychological ones. I looked for signs of depression, but saw none. Because I had worked so hard to prepare him for this illness, I was happy that I saw no adverse psychological effects. Perhaps Charles had finally realized that I had other things to do and was not there just for him. He realized, before I did, that I wasn't really there for him as I should have been.

Luckily for Charles, not long after the mood changes became apparent, his episode of Guillian-Barré started resolving. He was over the hill; the worse was behind him. The syndrome was leaving his body and now he could start planning for recuperation. But recovery would not occur before his body metamorphosis. His full face was drawn and pale. His once well-built frame mutated into a withered skeleton. His strong muscles had disappeared beneath the sheets of his hospital bed. He was now a thin, pale, weak physical being. His movement returned, slowly and conversely to the weakening sequence. He first regained movement of his upper body followed by his lower extremities. As his muscle strength returned, we were able to wean him off the ventilator support and allow the tracheostomy to heal. Daily physical therapy sessions helped reverse the muscle atrophy as Charles prepared for his transition to the extended care facility for additional rehabilitation.

His emotional psyche never returned to where it was as he rolled into our unit. He did remain unbelievably hardy despite my attempts to enforce my own need on him. I know now that I had prepared Charles for this journey, then I let him down by imposing my own needs on him. He was the patient, he was the one in need, he was depending on me to take care of him and I tried my hardest to do it at my convenience, not his.

Looking back, I realize I made Charles into the dependent person he became. I also look back at my own behavior and see that I was at fault. I am ashamed of my behavior when I think of how I really did neglect him by not attending to his calls. I became a nurse to help others, to care for them, to provide a service. What happened with Charles is that I developed a relationship with him, established trust that I would be there for him, and then when it was no longer convenient for me, I let him down. I shutter when I think of what I would need if I were in his condition. I dread the thought that I, too, may someday be helpless and in need of attention. When I rethink this experience, I realize that it was my immaturity, in my early nursing years, which fueled that unfortunate need to be in control despite the needs of my patient.

* * *

I've learned a lot since Charles. I have grown, matured, and hopefully I am wiser now. More recently I had another patient similar to Charles. Unlike Charles' temporary situation that resulted in a lack of communication, this patient was dealing with a permanent problem.

Jim was a 54-year-old man, suffering from Amyotrophic Lateral Sclerosis (ALS). ALS is a degenerative disease that affects the spinal cord. ALS is also known as Lou Gehrig's disease because of the famous baseball player who died from this disease. ALS results in a chronic debilitating state of weakness where the victim looses the ability to control his muscles. End-stage ALS finds the victim bedridden, with no control of their limp body, but totally intact cognitively. The mind is totally intact, but the body is useless.

Jim had been diagnosed with ALS several years prior to this admission. He was becoming weaker and weaker over the past few years, but he had continued to maintain some independence. Getting around in a wheelchair and the help from his wife allowed him to move from chair to bed to bathroom and back again. Until recently, he had been home with his wife, living a somewhat normal life. Six weeks prior to admission, Jim became ill with a minor cold. A simple illness that many of us could fight off resulted in a devastating turn of events for Jim and his wife. Because of his debilitative disease, a cold had resulted a six-week hospital stay requiring ventilator support and a new tracheostomy. After the acute event, Jim was weaned off the ventilator, and transferred to an extended care facility for further care. Even though Jim was no longer ventilator dependent, the tracheostomy was left in place to help ease his work of breathing. Two weeks of rehabilitation and therapy helped Jim recuperate and regain his independence. It was decided that Jim was ready to go back home with his attentive wife.

Jim's wife was excited to have him home again, but the excitement quickly evolved into anxiety. His recent illness had taken a toll on his strength, and resulted in a more debilitated state for Jim.

He was home only a few days when his weakened respiratory muscles caused him to be so short of breath that his wife brought him to our hospital.

After being examined in the emergency department, Jim was admitted to the hospital. He was weak; the past few months had resulted in a significant deterioration of his strength. Tracheotomy intact, Jim was showing signs of respiratory distress and was easily attached to the ventilator for support. The ventilator would help decrease the effort required to breathe. With the changes in his condition, his physician decided to provide the support for his respiratory muscles that he could no longer provide for himself. Jim was admitted to ICU to receive the ventilator support he needed.

The first day I cared for Jim, he was on the ventilator with moderate support. He was receiving intravenous fluids in addition to being fed through a feeding tube that had previously been inserted directly into his stomach. He had already spent two days in the ICU. His doctor had ordered ventilator support as needed. A routine had been established and Jim was attached to the ventilator only at night. During the day, he was left to breath on his own with some supportive oxygen. His respiratory status had stabilized, but the trach would now be permanent. If, at the end of this hospitalization, Jim did not need continuous ventilator support, he would still have quick access, using his trach, to ventilator support if needed. Most likely, due to the ALS, Jim would be ventilator dependent for the remainder of his life.

As I entered the room I saw a healthy looking man. His skin color was pink, not the usual paleness of most of my patients. He had a smile on his face that greeted me as I entered his room, along with his bright and shinning eyes. My first impression as I strolled cautiously into his domain, was that he was not a man that was going to let anything get him down. Despite the events of the past six weeks, he was still displaying this illuminated face.

I went about my business: completing my assessment, monitoring the machinery, checking the feeding pump, and double checking the settings on the ventilator. I reviewed the plan of care for the day. We would take him off the ventilator, monitor him closely, and at any time he felt he needed help breathing, we would reconnect him to his machine.

Communication with Jim was a challenge. The trach eliminated any possibility of sound, so lip reading was the next option. Because intubated patients are common in the ICU, lip reading is an easily acquired skill. I claim to be rather proficient in this skill and often am called upon by my co-workers to tell them what their patients are saying. Lip reading with Jim, I quickly realized, was going to be a problem. Within the first few sentences, it was evident that his ALS had also affected the muscles of his mouth and lips. Of course, I should have figured that when I was told he already had the gastric feeding tube in place. Gastric feeding tubes are inserted when patients cannot chew and swallow. Chewing and swallowing requires muscle control. Talking and forming words, requires muscle control as well. Jim's lips did not close; they never touched each other. His tongue was weak and ineffective. He was mouthing words to me with very little tongue movement and never closing his lips. Even though I repeatedly asked him to say things again and again, he never showed frustration. I found an alphabet board that immediately became our best friend. As I pointed to the correct letter, he would raise his eyebrow in approval. We spelled key words, using the alphabet board and we seemed to meet his needs with fewer hurdles.

Communicating with Jim was a time consuming adventure. Never could I enter the room, have a "conversation," and retreat within a few minutes. When reading those lazy lips did not work, out came the board. Because of Jim's limited movement, he also had no way of getting my attention. Unlike Charles, Jim could not snap his tongue when he needed me. He could not even shake his head to get my attention. The only movement Jim had to offer was his eyes and limited lip movement. I learned quickly that I always needed to look at Jim before leaving the room to see if he had anything else to say.

Communicating with Jim, while in the room, was challenging, but still possible. Communicating with Jim when I was not in the room proved to be impossible. All patients in the hospital have some type of call system. The most popular call bells are attached to the wall with a cord. The other end of the cord is located close to the bed so the patients can call for help using a hand-held device. The device has a button that the patient pushes that activates either a light and/or a bell.

The problem is, these call bells were developed for patients who can push a button. That's nice, but some patients cannot push a button. Alternative style call bells have been developed for those who cannot push that important button. These devices have a pad rather than a button. The pad can be positioned in the bed, next to the patient, and the patient can use gross movement of arms or elbows to tap the pad resulting in the bell activation. For those who do not have any movement below the neck, the call pad can be placed next to the head. Activation is then possible when the patient turns his head to the side to apply pressure on the pad and activates the call.

In Jim's room, one of the previous nurses had dutifully obtained this alternative call pad. Someone was assuring that Jim had the tool he needed for help. Unfortunately, in addition to his body weakness, Jim had limited movement of his head. The generalized weakness that had overcome his entire body also included his head, which prevented him from being able to adequately use this call pad. What the nurse didn't know about Jim was that like other ALS patients, he did still have more controlled movement of his feet. But this call pad was not at the foot of the bed; it was at the head of the bed, the area where he had less control.

I remembered another ALS patient I had cared for in the past. He, too, was cared for at home; he, too, was ventilator dependent; and he, too, had more movement of his feet than he did of his head. I remembered the other patient's wife had invented a call system for her husband that was unique to his needs. She had attached a bell to a string and then to a helium balloon. The balloon floated to the ceiling and the string was long enough to hold the bell just above the bed covers. The balloon and the bell were positioned at the foot of the bed. As he wiggled his toes, the bell would ring. This provided that patient the ability to use his last functioning movement to call for help.

It didn't take me long to determine that this call pad, attached to the head of the bed, was not going to be the best option for Jim. Even if he could use his head to push the pad, that was only an option when it was within reach to his head. For any of us who have spent any time in the hospital, we know that those beds have the capability to bend in the middle and raise the head of the bed. This is great for comfort, but the problem is, the nurses are always pulling the patient up in the bed. We pull them up, raise the head of the bed, and it's no time before they slide down again. Gravity required the nurses to pull those patients up again and again. For Jim, as he slid down in the bed, the call pad became inaccessible. The previous nurse had diligently thought of the call pad, but she failed to think of a way to keep it directly next to Jim.

I could see that this system was not going to work for Jim. With the memories of the helium balloon, I asked him if it was easier to move his feet than it was to move his head.

He nodded, a weak movement, in agreement.

So, at that time I decided action was necessary. The cord of the call pad was attached to the wall at the head of the bed, like everything else. Because of the layout of our ICU, all machines, pumps, and equipment that require any electrical support must be attached to that same wall at the head of the bed.

I pulled the cord of the call pad to the foot of the bed. Not surprisingly, I found that the cord was too short to reach the other end of the bed. Get an extension cord—not a possibility for this type of apparatus. Plug it into another place—not an option for any cord in the ICU. Since I could not get the call pad to the foot of the bed, I would have to get the foot of the bed to the call pad.

I decided to rearrange the room. This is not a common action. The equipment is all positioned on one wall and the head of the bed is always positioned on that same wall. That's just how it is. But for Jim, just because it's always that way, was not going to be good enough for him. I unlocked the wheels, pushed the head of the bed to the right, over to the sidewall and swung the foot of the bed toward the opposite wall. I left space on the right side of the room, at the head of the bed for the nurses to get around to the cardiac monitor. I left space on the left side of the room for all other activities. Finally, I suspended the cord of the call pad through the air and draped it over the foot of the bed. Threading the cord through the end and hanging the pad against the foot of the bed allowed for Jim to tap the pad with little movement of his foot.

"Can you reach that?" I asked.

A movement of his foot demonstrated his ability to tap the pad.

"Do you think that will work?" I knew the answer before I asked that one.

His smile told me all I needed to know. Words were not necessary for our communication at that moment.

I continued to rearrange his IV pump, his feeding pump, and I positioned the currently unused ventilator on the side of the bed. The room wasn't in the normal, orderly arrangement, but it was in the arrangement that was necessary for this patient. Normal position of the bed wasn't suitable because the normal call system was not workable for him. It was arranged in a way that was necessary for Jim to call for help. It was an arrangement that was necessary for this patient to get what he needed and deserved.

Jim and I enjoyed our day. Each of us has a favorite professional baseball team from the area. They were playing against each other on TV, and I was able to tease him when "my team" beat "his team." I took time to communicate with him while in the room, and he was able to maintain independence enough to call me when I was not there.

The next day, when I returned to work, I entered the room as I was receiving report, and the first thing I saw was that same call pad, again positioned at the head of his bed. The bed was neatly positioned perpendicular to the wall with all the outlets. Jim had slid down in bed, and the call pad was at least six inches above his head.

"How is he supposed to use that?" I asked the previous nurse, pointing to the useless pad.

"Oh, he always slips down in bed," was her uncaring response.

"I had that at the foot of the bed yesterday." I was trying to identify if there might be a good reason it was back in that useless position.

"The ventilator wouldn't reach him with his head over there." She pointed to the other wall. "We had to pull the bed back."

As I looked behind the ventilator, I noticed several yards of cords coiled up behind the machine. It was obvious to me that the convenient thing to do was to move the bed, rather than the ventilator and the other machines in the room. I politely reminded the nurse going off duty that Jim didn't have much movement of his head, and the movement of his feet allowed him to call for help when needed. As quickly as our morning report was finished, I encouraged her to leave the room and go home, before I lost my temper. I had taken extra steps to provide the best way for him to communicate. I had made sure his call system worked for him. I had established a method for Jim to alert the nurses when he needed help. She had undone all my efforts with one quick sweep of the bed.

I looked into Jim's appealing eyes as he opened his mouth. His entire mouth was full of saliva, saliva that may have been collecting for hours. Jim had been unable to call for help and had been required to hold that saliva in his mouth until someone conveniently entered the room. As I suctioned the abundance of liquid from his mouth, I found myself wanting to apologize for what the other nurse had, or had not done. I found myself getting frustrated, that what I had worked so hard to orchestrate the previous day had been undone. I was worried that Jim had not received the tools he needed to communicate all night long. Without the call button at the foot of the bed, Jim was at the mercy of the nurse to care for him when she thought he needed it, not at the moment when he really wanted it.

I could only imagine what Jim was thinking. Was he glad to have me there at that moment? Was he glad to have his mouth clean? Was he going to have to rush through all his needs in order to get them met while I was in the room because as soon as I left, he was at my mercy for when I decided he might need some more assistance? I could see it in his eyes, he was grateful for what I was doing, but he still didn't have complete faith in me.

It didn't take long to change the expression on Jim's face. And it didn't take long to rearrange that room once again. This time I not only repositioned the bed to the side of the room, but I put the ventilator over there too. I took a big piece of tape and secured the cord of the call pad to the foot of the bed, and I placed a big sign at the head of the bed requesting all staff to keep the call pad on the foot of the bed. Now I could see, through the expressions in his eyes, that he knew I would be there for him, when he needed me, not at my convenience, but when he actually called.

Every day when I cared for Jim, he was able to call when he needed me. The arrangement of the room was a small inconvenience that was required to allow him to maintain his independence. Those small inconveniences allowed Jim to get the care he deserved—when he needed it. Those same inconveniences allowed Jim to have a good experience in our ICU.

* * *

I now know that communication is a basic necessity for all, especially those patients in ICU who have multiple, complex needs. Many of our patients have limited means of communication. By taking their voice away, or limiting their movement, we restrict their ability to call for help in many ways. Communication is vital for our patient to get what they need and deserve.

As I look back at these two situations—one early in my nursing career and the other more recent—I see how I have grown, how I have realized that these patients need me to be there for them—when they need me, not when I want them to need me. I have let go of some control and relinquished it to my patients. They are the ones in need, not me. My patients have the right to express their desires. They have the right to communicate their needs, and I am there to provide that service for them. When the nurse undid what I had done for Jim, I assumed she had taken the easy way out, and not wanted to be bothered. I apologized for what she had done. I wish Charles were here now so I could apologize for taking the easy way out and not wanting to be bothered and for what I had done to him, many years ago.

The ICU nurse accepts responsibility to care for critically ill patients. The patients in the ICU need more attention, which is why they are placed in this area. The nurse must make herself available to her patients at all times, not just when it is convenient. She must be there for *all* of their needs, *when* they need her. Working in the ICU is a fast paced, high level of nursing, and the nurse must be willing to provide a fast paced, high level of care at all times.

Not What You Think

One morning I was receiving report from the night shift charge nurse. At change of shift, there is a report from charge nurse to charge nurse, in order to relay any pertinent information that needs to be pursued. This report occurs simultaneously with the individual reports that each nurse is receiving at the bedside. As I was receiving report, one of the nurses from the night shift entered the room. He, the male nurse, apologized for interrupting the important exchange of information, but continued on to declare that he had some urgent information. As he approached, I noticed that his left hand remained gloved. It's not good nursing practice to walk around the unit with gloved hands. Gloves are removed as soon as the task is complete and just prior to hand washing. Not only did he still have the glove on, but also he was carrying a bedpan in that gloved hand. And, that bedpan was not empty. Why was he bringing a bedpan into the report room?

Upon entering, he immediately started explaining why he was presenting this excrement to the charge nurse. "I just want to make sure you see what my patient did." He explained, as he presented the bedpan within easy view of us both. "My patient has been constipated for the past three days, and I am such a good nurse, I was able to help him accomplish the difficult task of moving his bowels."

I still was not sure why he needed to bring this to the attention of the charge nurses. As I grimaced and leaned in the opposite direction of the disgusting presentation, he continued. "You need to see this." He paused briefly, "These small stools are perfectly shaped."

36

I couldn't help but to wonder, what was so impressive about a few small turds in a bedpan? We see that everyday.

"Each one of them is the same shape, and almost the same size too," he continued.

Now I was wondering about his sanity.

"They don't even smell bad." With this, he was trying to shove them toward my face, but I instinctively moved further away. I didn't need to smell what was in that bedpan. I could see those small brown deposits that he was so proud of.

"And believe it or not, they don't taste bad either." His words and his motions were simultaneous. As he picked up one of those small soft brown logs and placed it in his mouth, I could not believe my eyes.

He instantaneously started chewing and laughing at the same time. Now with the smell of his breath, I too started laughing. I smelled chocolate. But I stopped laughing long enough to threaten to assault him for making me think that he had lost his mind. He could barely stop laughing long enough to explain how he so delicately half chewed a few small brownies, shaped them into the appropriate size and shapes and carefully positioned them in a perfectly clean bedpan, next to a clean crinkled piece of toilet tissue. He did all this, just to play a practical joke on some unsuspecting, naive charge nurses.

CHAPTER 4

Code Blue

What really happens during a Code Blue?
How the ICU team works to save lives.

"Code Blue" is the announcement made when a patient has a cardiac or respiratory arrest. I often joke with the newer, inexperienced nurses about becoming wallpaper when they encounter their first Code Blue. Wallpaper sticks to the wall, does nothing, and no one really notices it. I too was wallpaper at one time. It's only with experience that each of us becomes more comfortable with these emergency situations, but never comfortable with the outcome that so often occurs.

* * *

I was young and inexperienced when I started my career on a medical floor. I had only been working for about a year, when one day I entered a four-bed ward of male patients. I was bringing in a lunch tray for Mr. Murphy. He was 78-years-old and recuperating from pneumonia.

Suddenly I noticed Mr. Murphy wasn't recuperating as well as he should be. His skin was no longer pink, his raspy voice was silent, and his slightly labored breathing had disappeared. Mr. Murphy lay lifeless in his bed. His eyes were slightly sunken and almost closed, as if he was peeking out under his soft eyelids. His cheeks were ashen gray, not the pale pink they were just moments ago when I gave his roommates their lunch. And his lips were as blue as the ocean water at sunset.

"Mr. Murphy," I yelled, as I almost threw his lunch on the floor.

"Mr. Murphy," I screeched once again as I shook his shoulder and pleaded in my own mind. *Please don't let this be happening, just a few minutes ago, you smiled at me as I left the room.*

Oh no, what now. The thoughts were racing through my head. *Run for help, no stay right here, this was my responsibility. Flatten the bed, call a Code Blue, pull the curtains so the others in the room won't see, start CPR.* All these ideas were scrambled in my thoughts, while what I really wanted to do was turn around, walk away, and come back into the room all over again. Maybe the next time, he would be smiling again and this would have been just a bad dream. No, this time it was for real.

As I lowered the head of the bed flat, I kept calling his name and shaking his shoulder. I was hoping by some miracle he would open his eyes and take that breath that he had forgotten to take. Mr. Murphy was not going to help me, so it was my job to help him. The Code Blue bell was buzzing in the distant background, but it seems like the clock was ticking at a snail's pace. *Where were the others? This was supposed to be a team effort, teamwork, team nursing; I learned that in school. Where was my charge nurse, who was supposed to help me with stressful situations? Where was the crash cart with all the tools and equipment we needed to save lives? Where was the doctor who went to school a lot longer than I did and gets paid a lot more than I do to perform these kinds of tasks.*

At that moment, it was only me, so I did what I was taught to do. Taught from a book, this was not something we practiced in the nursing skills lab. Unlike giving each other shots, there were no nursing students who would volunteer to stop breathing so the classmates could practice bringing them back to life. I was taught to hyperextend the head and lift the chin to open the airway. Look at the chest to see if it was rising—was air entering the chest? Position my ear just above the face to listen for any sounds—sounds that may indicate any signs of breathing. And, finally keep my face close to his, to feel for any air movement.

Nothing, nothing was happening, no movement of the chest, no air flowing in or out of the mouth or nose. For God sake, this man was not breathing. This was what I went to school for, to help sick people. But, I was the only one there now. I was his only hope. Practice or not, it was time to save my first life.

I placed my mouth over the cold, wet, limp lips of Mr. Murphy. My mouth sunk into his lifeless cheeks as I created an airtight seal around his mouth. I blew life into his cool, pale body. Not once, but twice, just as I was taught to do. Two deep breaths. As I held back the waves of nausea that had suddenly come over me, I slid my right hand down to his neck to check for a pulse. I held firm pressure on the carotid artery located on the front of his neck, hoping that there would be some sign of life. I was hoping—please let me feel some weak pulsation under my fingertips. No, nothing there either, so I climbed onto the bed with Mr. Murphy. I held back the waves of nausea caused by his cold, wet, sullen lips. I needed to position myself above him in order to lean over his body and start chest compressions. The bed was too high. I didn't have a stool to raise myself up so I climbed onto the bed. I knelt with my knees against his ribs, positioned my hands on the lower end of his sternum, the breastbone, and pushed as hard as I could. Now that I had breathed what little air I had into his lungs, I needed to circulate it to his vital organs. Without oxygen, this man would never be smiling at anyone again.

One, two, three, compressions. It was now my job to squeeze his heart between the breastbone and the backbone to push the blood through the blood vessels so it could travel out to the entire body. Four, five ... Oh, thank God, the team finally arrived. The 240-pound orderly took over the job of chest compressions. His strong arms would surely be more effective in circulating the blood than mine. The respiratory therapist entered with mask and ambu bag in hand. He slipped the mask onto Mr. Murphy's face, attached the ambu bag to the oxygen and squeezed air into those empty oxygen-starved lungs.

I backed off, away from the bed, watching the team function like a finely tuned orchestra. Each member did the job they were assigned. The physician took charge of medications, airway management, and leadership; the respiratory therapist provided breaths and oxygenation; the orderly compressed the chest for effective circulation; and the code nurse gave the emergency medications—as instructed by the physician—that would bring life back to this lovely gentleman who was, just moments ago, smiling at his young, inexperienced nurse.

As the code team did their job, I sank into the surroundings, still trying to fight back the nausea and now also fighting back the tears that would sneak from my innocent eyes as I watched my first patient die. I became the wallpaper on the walls of that cold hospital room. Like wallpaper, I wanted to blend into the walls so no one would notice me. I wasn't sure I wanted to be noticed. I wasn't sure I wanted to be in that room. I wasn't even sure if I wanted to work in this career that experiences death day after day. Those were normal feelings for the young, inexperienced nurse. That's probably why young, inexperienced nurses are not on the Code Blue team.

* * *

The Code Blue team, just about every hospital has one, is a team of experienced staff who can take charge of emergency medical situations. Each hospital may call it something different and have a different combination of people, but the goal is the same. These are the people who will respond to emergencies, take charge, do what is best for the patient, and try their hardest to save lives.

The physician will take charge at the head of the bed. He enters the room, immediately starts asking questions. Who is the patient? Why is he/she in the hospital? What happened before the event? The physician asks the pertinent questions to gather valid information and takes charge of the situation. As he positions himself at the head of the bed, his first action is to secure an airway for the patient in the bed who is not breathing.

The respiratory therapists, who usually arrive in pairs, are responsible for the airway and oxygenation. They work in tandem, one opening the airway while the other secures the oxygen. They place a mask on the face of the patient, one holding securely with two strong hands, while the other squeezes air into the lungs with the ambu-bag. All this, while simultaneously assisting the physician in the preparation for the insertion of an artificial airway into the lungs in order to breath for another human being.

The orderlies, those wonderful strong people who roam the halls helping move, lift, walk, and transport the patients, enter with the team to provide the chest compressions. Again, just like in Noah's Ark, there are two. The first will take over compressions from the poor nurse who found this lifeless body, while the second stands back waiting for the first to tire out. These two rescuers take turns doing the chest compressions, one relieving the other, for the entire time of the Code Blue.

The nurses, frequently two of them, are often from the emergency department, or the ICU. The first steps into the role of the medication nurse, assuring there is an intravenous line to administer medications. Having access to the tray of emergency medications, she will inject the medications at the directions of the physician. Without medications, successful recessitation is not likely.

The second RN becomes the team leader; it will be her job to keep control of the highly volatile, stressful situation. She oversees the entire orchestra, making sure each section performs as needed. She pulls equipment out of the crash cart that has been delivered to the room specifically for this event. A tower of drawers supplied with IV's, tubings, needles, and medications, hopefully everything that will be needed. She draws blood, labels it and hands it to whomever is staring at her, waiting to run the specimen to the lab so the team can get vital information about why their victim was not doing what we all want him/her to do. That would of course be, to live. The team leader also provides crowd control, sending the third and fourth respiratory therapist out of the room, sending the extra orderlies out of the room, and shooing away all the other nurses, pharmacists, managers, who just happen to be walking down the hall at the time of the announcement. And, finally, the team leader is the one, now that she is experienced, who will keep this patient's nurse from becoming wallpaper. This patient's nurse must now become part of this team, whether she wants to or not. That nurse is the one who will provide the facts, the fragmented pieces of information, that will help the physician decipher what is happening to the patient, and what we, as a team must do to keep the patient alive.

* * *

I will never forget my first code, the nausea, the fright, and the tears of disappointment. Now, many years later, the nausea and fright are gone, but often the tears of disappointment are still there. Sometimes disappointment that we brought the poor soul back to life, and sometimes disappointment that we did not.

* * *

George came to our hospital in the winter. Fifty-eight-years-old, George had been institutionalized and bed-ridden for almost twenty years with multiple sclerosis. Multiple Sclerosis (MS) is a chronic, progressive disease of the central nervous system that causes muscle weakness, often resulting in total paralysis. In addition to muscle weakness, MS may result in mental deterioration towards the end of the illness. George came to our acute facility when he developed an infection in his bedsores. On that cold winter day when George was admitted to the ICU, his temperature was 102 degrees and he was having difficulty breathing. George was thin, even though he was being fed through a tube inserted through his abdomen, directly into his stomach. A high-calorie formula was pumped into his stomach to provide the exact amount of calories to sustain life. Now that George had an infection, we would increase the number of calories to assure he had additional energy to fight his illness. George didn't talk to us; he didn't speak. There were no facial expressions to let us know what he wanted or needed. He did open his eyes and sometimes looked around at his surroundings. However, he never did acknowledge us by looking into our eyes or gazing in our direction. George didn't move, unless we moved him. He just lay in the bed, contracted, his elbows no longer extended because the muscles in his arms had atrophied. His legs were curled up like a babies, hips contracted, knees contracted, all the muscles shortened due to lack of use. He was not able to communicate or move, and totally dependent on us for all of his bodily needs. We cared for him, treated his fever, tended to his respiratory distress, and gave him antibiotics to cure the infection.

At the time of admission, the doctors initiated a conversation with George's family. As with most patients in ICU, the doctors, and sometimes the nurses, initiate the discussion about end-of-life choices. Very old, very ill, or chronically ill patients often do not want life-sustaining treatment. Quality of life is often a determining factor in decisions. Those who can no longer live what they consider a quality life may choose not to prolong death. We, the healthcare providers, do everything we can to cure the current illness, but in the event of cardiopulmonary arrest, we need to establish if the patient wants us to do CPR and call a Code Blue. In this case, since George could not communicate, and his sister had a durable power of health care for him, the discussion was held with the sister. She assured us that she wanted everything done, at all costs, to save George's life.

After his infection was cured, George was ready to go back to his nursing home. But this time it wasn't so easy. George's pressure ulcers, commonly called bedsores, were still rather extensive and required ongoing treatment. The nursing home would not admit patients with pressure ulcers that required complicated dressing changes. Even though these ulcers developed while George was a resident at that same nursing home, it was their policy that no patient would be admitted with complicated wounds. George had enjoyed a stay at our hospital long enough to qualify as a new admission to his old nursing home.

There was one minor problem that would prevent him from returning to the home he had known for almost twenty years. That one minor problem was two craters, the size of my fist, on each of his hips. His wounds were our main concern now. We provided him with a special mattress, not a normal mattress like you or I would have if we came to the hospital. His special mattress was filled with sand, and when plugged into the wall, air would flow and George would float on the sand mattress like a pillow. We cleaned and dressed the wounds twice a day. Two nurses spent almost an hour, removing dressings, cleaning the wounds, and repacking the clean crevices. We kept George in the ICU for many weeks because of the labor intensive dressing changes. The procedure was too time consuming for the medical floor nurses. They could not take the necessary time from their team of patients. So we, the ICU nurses, were the only hope George had to getting back to his home, as he knew it. It was up to us, to heal these wounds and send him home.

Several weeks later, the wounds were healing, slowly of course, and the dressings were finally at the point where the medical floor nurse could accommodate George on their unit. Despite the fact that the wounds were healing, it was evident that this illness had taken a toll on George's emaciated body. He was thinner; despite the high calorie formula we were feeding him. He never opened his eyes any more. He was withering away in that luxury sand bed. As we prepared George for transfer to the medical floor, we reviewed all his orders. Once again we spoke to the sister about end-of-life decisions—the sister who rarely came to visit. Our only contact with her was by phone; we would leave a message and she would call back at her convenience. Once contacted, she assured us she wanted everything done to keep her debilitated brother alive. So we honored her wishes. We continued to provide the high standard of care as we had been. We continued to care for those atrocious wounds, and hoped to get George back to his nursing home. Late in the evening he was transferred to the medical floor, and that's the last we heard about George ... for a while.

* * *

One summer morning, several months after George left our unit, I was assigned as the charge nurse. One of the duties of the charge nurse was to respond to all Code Blue calls throughout the hospital. Just as I was beginning my own rounds, "Code Blue" was announced three times over the public administration system, as it always was. The room number was announced and I went running. Up the elevator, several floors up, the Code Blue team was activated.

As I arrived in the room, everyone was dressing in gowns and masks. This patient had an infection that shouldn't be spread. I dressed in my gown, mask and gloves, on the move as I entered the room. Surprisingly I saw George, lying there pale, cold, and lifeless. Months had passes since he came to us for help. His extended stay had allowed George to make this his new home. Now something had suddenly changed. The bedside nurse was trying to tell anyone in the room who would listen, what she had found. She just finished getting report from the previous nurse, she came into the room to take his vital signs before breakfast and found him. Pale blue, cold and clammy, and barely breathing. His chest was practically still, but his neck muscles showed signs of respiratory efforts.

Within seconds, the entire Code Blue team had arrived. The physician quickly inserted the tube into his lungs to establish an airway. The orderly was providing strong chest compressions. The emergency room nurse was administering the required medications. I assumed the team leader role, while everyone was waiting to see how strong George really was.

First round of drugs were given.

"Stop CPR, check a pulse," demanded the physician.

"No pulse," reported the orderly.

We continued CPR and administered another round of drugs. Epinephrine, Atropine, and this time we even tried some Sodium

Bicarbonate to fight off acidosis that occurs during cardiac arrest. The nurse manager phoned George's sister to inform her of the change in condition. She made sure she knew that her brother had had a cardiac arrest and we were working hard to bring him back to life. Many family members will rush to the hospital when informed of this type of emergency. Most want a chance to see their loved ones, one last time. George's sister gave no verbal indication that she was coming, "Just be sure you call my Mom," was her request. She wanted the manager to call her estranged mother and give her the same information that she had just heard. The team continued to work hard to save George's life; another round of medications, continuous CPR, followed by another pulse check. We still had no luck when searching for a pulse that would indicate signs of life. We had been trying to resuscitate George for what seemed like an eternity.

"Stop CPR, let's call the code," instructed the emergency physician.

Call the code, which means all members are to stop their efforts. This was done when the Code Blue was unsuccessful, the patient had not responded, death had occurred. The team had not done what they set out to do. This time we did not save the life, or did we?

The physician looked around the room seeing all the team members pulling back. The orderly had stopped doing chest compressions. The nurse had stopped administering medications and had turned off the IV's. The respiratory therapist had stopped bagging air into his lungs. With the doctor's hand on George's groin, feeling for a femoral pulse, he said to the respiratory therapist who remained at the head of the bead.

"I don't feel a pulse, do you?"

She hesitated, with wide eyes, and responded while holding her hand on the carotid artery, "Yes, I do."

The physician quickly reaches for the side of the neck and palpated a slow weak movement beneath his fingers.

"Restart the IV's, give another ampule of Epinephrine, and check his blood pressure," he commanded the team back into action.

George was once again, showing us how strong he was. The code team kick started their actions all over again. This time they hung bags of medications that would increase George's blood pressure. With the addition of the new artificial support, we could now call our efforts successful.

George was transported to the ICU after the Code Blue, as all patients are. All the nurses remembered him. "Poor George" was what most of them were saying. "Poor George," because now he couldn't go on to a bright new home in the sky; we pulled him back. "Poor George," would continue to wither away in that luxury sand bed; loosing weight despite our efforts to nourish him, contracting into a ball despite our limb exercises. "Poor George," would have to remain here on earth with us, alone.

George remained with us in ICU only for a few more hours. Despite the continuous infusion of medications to support his blood pressure, later that day the Code Blue team was activated once again. When George's pulse faded away the next time, the code team was unable to bring him back for another rally. That next time, George was finally able to move beyond our efforts and move onto his new home, in the sky.

The nurses were not sad that George died that day. Some were actually glad, relieved that George would not have to suffer any longer. We knew that the only life George had was to lie in that sand bed, depend on others for every aspect of care, and not be able to communicate, eat, or enjoy life. After many years of lingering illness, George was at peace. It was time for George to move on to a better place.

Sometimes we announce a Code Blue because we are required to save the life, despite our beliefs that that person would be happy to be left undisturbed. Often because of family constraints, we code patients and do CPR even if we know in our hearts that it's not the right thing to do. Prolonging suffering and illness that prevents any human being from being a human being may not be the best choice; but for us, it is the only choice. Sometimes the Code Blue is successful, and sometimes it's not. Some would say Georges' last Code Blue was not successful because he died, but for some we would say it was.

∗ ∗ ∗

Claire was not alone in her journey. Claire had a close, supportive family—six children, and even more grandchildren. Claire came to our ICU one morning after I received a call from the manager of the surgical floor.

"I have a patient who doesn't look good." Those were her nonspecific instructions as to why that patient needed to be transferred to the ICU.

That's often how the floor nurses start the conversation when they call ICU about a patient. They think that will get them a bed in our busy ICU.

"I don't have a nurse to take care of this one, " was my first response. "What's wrong with her?"

The manager continued to inform me that this eighty-eight-year-old lady was doing fine yesterday. Today she was in a lot of pain and despite being on a non-rebreather mask—that administers a hundred percent oxygen—she was having difficulty breathing and maintaining a sufficient oxygen level.

"Have you called the Rapid Response Team?" I asked, in an attempt to delay her. I was hoping the Rapid Response Team would be able to initiate some interventions that might stabilizer her. And that might postpone or even prevent her transfer to ICU.

The manager agreed to initiate a call. But meanwhile, I went to bed 8 and got the area ready. Just in case they have to bring this patient to the ICU, and take my only empty bed, I would prepare the area. I made sure all the equipment was stocked, and brought the paperwork to the bedside. Sometimes I'm a little superstitious. I think if I prepare for the admissions, they might not come. This time I would be ready and hope she didn't have to come.

Within minutes, Claire was being pushed through the door. The Rapid Response Team didn't buy me enough time to get another nurse to take care of this patient. Now she was in my ICU and I would be her nurse, along with my charge nurse duties. As she rolled in, I saw a frail, pale little old lady who reminded me of my own mother-in-law. I quickly learn that she had had surgery a week ago. Originally, she came to the hospital with abdominal pain, spent several days being worked up by a variety of physicians, and finally, one week ago, surgery was performed. Claire had a history of chronic obstructive pulmonary disease (COPD). Initially after surgery, she came to ICU for a few days and was on a ventilator, commonly referred to as life support. After being weaned off the ventilator, and recovering on schedule, she was transferred out of ICU, to the surgical floor. Her family told me that yesterday she was doing well. She was out of bed, walking, and even started eating. They were anticipating her discharge within a few days.

Today she was short of breath, in a lot of pain, and was just "not right." A few of the family members remained with her as I settled her into her ICU bed. This family was not going anywhere. They were genuinely concerned, and waiting for something to be done.

I started my assessment. Her blood pressure was low, but the fluid bolus, which had been started upstairs, was just about finished. I heard wheezing sounds in her lungs so I asked for a respiratory treatment. And finally, I medicated her for her abdominal pain. After explaining everything to the family, I ask them if she had any end-of-life wishes.

"I know she was on a ventilator last week, was that something that she wants again if needed?" I needed to clarify her wishes and theirs.

"Yes, we want everything done," The son told me in a solemn voice.

I assured them that we were doing everything we needed to do. Her blood pressure was low, but we were giving her fluids. Her oxygen level was low, but we were giving her supplemental oxygen and breathing treatments. We would watch her closely, wait and see how she responded to the current interventions. The doctor would be coming soon, I reassured them.

Within an hour, her oxygen saturation, which we monitor with a light probe on the end of the finger, had increased from 93% to 100%. She looked better; I took the non-rebreather mask off and replaced it with a nasal cannula. She no longer needed 100% oxygen from the mask. The short oxygen prongs of the nasal cannula that sit gently in the nose are much more comfortable than a mask covering the entire face.

When the doctor came, he looked at me and said, "How's she doing?"

I reported that I had been able to wean her oxygen to a nasal cannula. Her oxygen saturation was 100% and her blood pressure was still low—92/48. She was still receiving fluids and had just received a dose of Morphine for pain but, overall she was feeling better.

He gave me orders to use whatever means of oxygen I needed to keep her oxygen saturation above 92%—then quickly asked me if the family still wanted everything done.

"Yes they do." I confirmed as I looked directly into the eyes of the son.

The doctor then looked at the son and asked, "Does she want to be put back on life support if she needs it?'

The puzzled look on the son's face initiated clarification.

"The ventilator," the doctor clarified.

"If that's what's needed." He shook his head affirmatively.

"O.K. I think we just dried her out too much. Let me know if anything changes." and off he went, out the door. By "dried her out," the doctor meant that the diuretics Claire had been given to rid her body of extra fluids, along with the fact that she had been eating and drinking very little, resulted in dehydration. Hopefully the fluids I was giving her would reverse this acute distress she was experiencing.

There I was, left caring for this poor little lady, while I was supposed to be in charge of the other twenty-eight patients and fourteen nurses. They're on their own for now. Each nurse would take charge of herself and the unit will have to run itself for now. Claire was my primary concern for this moment in time.

Over the next few hours, her oxygen saturation dropped slightly, 91%. I reinitiated oxygen therapy through a mask rather than just the nasal cannula. She didn't like the mask and kept taking it off to talk. So I kept the nasal prongs on, in addition to the mask, so she could take the mask off and still get supplemental oxygen. I reposition her, gave her sips of water, watched her falling urine output, all while continuing to give IV fluids. I kept hoping, once we got enough fluids in her system, that her urine output would increase, blood pressure would return to normal, and all would be well, once again.

At three o'clock, a float nurse was sent to my unit. Vicki was a medical nurse who sometimes floated into the ICU. She didn't work in ICU all the time, but had been oriented to the basic ICU skills. Just as I had done many years ago, Vicki would work in the ICU only when we didn't have enough of our regular staff. Just as I was dependent, many years ago, on the experienced ICU nurses to support me, she would depend on me to support her. She would relieve me of my assignment with Claire so I could once again take charge of the entire ICU.

Today, I especially appreciated that Vicki was willing to work outside her area. Now I could resume my charge nurse duties, but would make sure I was available to help and oversee the care that she would provide for this lovely little lady. I reported everything I knew about Claire. We discussed the plan of care. She would monitor the blood pressure, which was once again low after a second dose of Morphine. She would also watch the urine output that was dropping despite continued fluids. We discussed the need to call the doctor, inform him of Claire's status, and ask for a Dopamine drip. That would increase the blood pressure and hopefully help increase the urine output.

After speaking to the doctor, Vicki informed me that he had indeed given her an order to start Dopamine, but she didn't know how to start it. So I provided her with the clinical support she required and helped her with the care she was giving. Once again Claire's oxygen saturation was dropping. Now 90%, we decide to put her back on the non-rebreather mask that would deliver 100% oxygen.

As I was making rounds on all the other ICU patients, I was informed that despite the use of 100% oxygen, Claire's oxygen saturation was down in the 80's now. I could see that the oxygen mask was not doing what Claire needed. For some reason, she was not able to get enough oxygen. Another call to the doctor, another update, and another change in plans was needed. This time I coached Vicki to ask for an order for bi-pap. I knew this failing lady now needed ventilation support. Bi-pap—positive pressure mask—allows the patient to breath spontaneously with the support of additional pressure on each breath. As the patient takes a breath, the machine pushes with gentle pressure, to augment the shallow respirations. This positive pressure mask is a non-invasive form of ventilatory support. The full-face mask, positioned securely onto her face, would *push* oxygen into her lungs each time she took a breath. I could see the nurse who didn't normally work in this unit was a little uncertain. After reviewing her assessment of the patient, and assuring there were no other changes, I reiterated my instructions.

"Make sure you tell him that she is on the non-rebreather mask and her oxygen level is dropping. Tell him we want to start bi-pap." I remained face to face with her long enough to get a nod of understanding, and then I left her to do what I knew she could do.

Within a few minutes she was again at my side to let me know what she had accomplished. After relaying all of the information over the phone, the physician gave the order I wanted, for bi-pap. She had already called the respiratory therapist, and someone was on their way to initiate the treatment.

"Did he also give you an order to check ABG's?" I asked as I suddenly realized that I forgot to tell her that. I remembered, once again, that she didn't have the instinct and the experience that would have automatically made her ask for an order for follow-up ABG's when she asked for the bi-pap order.

"No, he only gave me the order for bi-pap." The look on her face insinuated that she had done something wrong.

"That's O.K. We'll start the bi-pap now, see how she does, and we'll get some ABG's if we need it."

I could tell by the look on her face, she was concerned that I was not following the doctor's order. With the uncertainty on her face, I explained that we have a protocol, standard of practice, that directs us to check ABG's a few hours after initiating bi-pap therapy in order to assure that the therapy is actually helping.

Just about that time, Claire's cardiologist came into the unit. He stopped by the bedside, checked on her, talked to the family for a few minutes, and then retreated to the nursing station to make a note in the chart.

"She has a weak heart, you know." He was giving me additional information that would help us care for Claire. How were we supposed to know how weak her heart was, except that it was eighty-eight-years-old.

"She's been through a lot for her age. Surgery always takes a lot out of old people." I wasn't sure if he was preparing himself or me for what might happen to Claire. As he and I were discussing her sequence of events, we suddenly noted that her heart rate was also changing. When she came to ICU earlier, her heart rate was 115 beats per minute. Then for a while she was running in the 90's, now her heart rate was in the 70's.

"I just don't feel good about this," I shared with him. "I hope the bi-pap works." We discussed the heart rate dropping, slowly over the last few hours. And we discussed the potential that Claire may need to be intubated and placed on a ventilator. We agreed that we did not want to wait for a code situation before intubating. We would initiate the bi-pap and watch her closely, for now. Before he left, to see the rest of his patients, we discussed the plan of care. Dopamine would be given for blood pressure support; bi-pap for breathing support, and a little TLC for family support. And, he gave me the order for the ABG's that I knew we would need to make sure that our newest intervention was working. At that time, it seemed like we were providing everything that Claire needed.

The family remained at the bedside throughout all of the changes; taking turns so we only had a few at a time. Each time we tried something different, we explained to Claire and her family. I explained that each time Claire took a breath; the bi-pap would push extra air into her lungs. We would watch her closely, give the bi-pap a chance, but if it didn't work, we would need to put her back on the breathing machine, like she was on a few days ago.

The eldest son gave a nod of approval, and I knew he understood this was now serious. Unfortunately, my next words were to explain the visiting restrictions. I had to request that the family leave the bedside because it was time for the nurses' shift change. The only time in our unit that the families are not allowed to visit was during shift change. We do this to maintain confidentiality while the nurses give report, at the bedside, to the next nurse.

As I was getting ready to give my own report to the charge nurse for the next shift, I walked past Claire's bed. I noticed her oxygen saturation was still 88% and now her heart rate was fluctuating between seventy-two and sixty-eight. Sixty-eight, too low, I didn't like that. It was continuing to drop and that was not right. I immediately went into my bossy charge nurse mode and I quickly demanded that Vicki call the doctor. "Tell him this bi-pap was not working and we needed to intubate Claire now." I was not going to wait to do ABG's, I could tell that the bi-pap was not reversing the untoward changes that I had seen over the last few hours.

"Should I tell him to call the emergency doctor?" she asks with her big eyes pleading for guidance.

"Tell him if he cannot be here in five minutes, I will call the emergency doctor myself."

I picked up another phone and called the respiratory therapists. "We need to intubate bed 8 now." My words went very forcefully through the hand receiver. I hung up the phone and went to the cupboard to get the intubation module. A small tray with sterile instruments used to insert a tube into the lungs.

As I walked back to Claire's bedside, I look up to the cardiac monitor—7:04—normal rhythm, narrow QRS complex. Then suddenly at 7:05, I saw the widening of the QRS complexes. Not only was the rate of the heart slowing, now the electrical conduction of the heart was slowing as well, a sign of lack of oxygen.

My thoughts started running rapidly through my head. *Oh no, she's going to die.* I wasn't going to wait five minutes; I wasn't going to wait to call the emergency doctor. I pushed the red button on the wall and, once again, the Code Blue team was activated.

This time I was already there and by some miracle, the respiratory therapist was right by my side. I ripped off the full-face mask, grabbed the ambu bag, placed the mask on her face, and lifted her chin. I was lifting the chin and hyper-extending the head. The respiratory therapist was squeezing the ambu bag but her chest was not rising. I lifted higher.

"Squeeze harder, the chest is not moving." I yelled.

Suddenly, we were surrounded by the Code Blue team and too many nurses. The emergency doctor arrived and I give him a brief background while he was moving in beside me at the head of the bed. He quickly intubated Claire with the tray that was placed on her chest for easy access.

With a squeeze of the ambu bag, the chest was now rising. Another squeeze, and air was heard in both lung fields on both sides of the chest.

Good work guys, we saved another one. Didn't even loose the pulse.

Just as we all took a breath, the cardiac monitor at the bedside displayed a surprise. Ventricular tachycardia, a life-threatening arrhythmia that quickly deteriorated to ventricular fibrillation. The heart was quivering now. Just as we, the code team, were feeling good about acting quickly, Claire threw us a curve ball.

The commands started. "Check a pulse." No pulse.

"Start CPR." The orderly moved into position.

"Shock her." We needed to shock this heart back into a normal rhythm.

"Give some Epinephrine." This is a drug to help stimulate the heart.

This time, the ICU charge nurse who had just started her shift took over as team leader. I retreated, moving away from the bed. Too many people create chaos, and that was not what was needed now.

Suddenly I found myself sliding into guilt feelings. I sent the family away, the family that had so dutifully sat next to the bed all day long. I sent them to the waiting room, away from their loved one. Now she was dying.

My guilt-ridden eyes capture the glance of the fresh charge nurse, the current team leader. "I'm going to talk to the family."

She nodded approval as I scurried for the door. Just outside the ICU door was our dreadful waiting room. Dreadful because what the family members use as a waiting room is a long hallway. Chairs lined up on one side, and a television sunken into the wall on the other. This hall is also the same hall our patients travel through coming and going from the ICU. A small room that seats only eight people, sits off to the side of the hallway. This private room gets evacuated on occasion to be used for family conferences and/or grieving families.

I glanced down the hall, I saw half a dozen family members, and none were Claire's. I turned to peek into the small room, more strangers looked back at me. I turned and looked again down the hall, still not there. *What have I done with them? Where have they gone? Don't they know "Code Blue" in ICU means they should come running back.* I would if my family was in ICU and I heard a "Code Blue" called. *Why did I send them away?* Because it was the rule, no visitors during shift change. Damn the rules. I should have known the bi-pap wasn't going to work. I should have told them to stay close so I could call them. I didn't know their mom would stop breathing at shift change. Now what?

Hurriedly I return to the ICU. "Overhead page the family," I barked to the unit secretary.

"Whom do you want?" she questions.

"I want the son and the granddaughter, they were just here," my voice was beginning to tremble. I could feel panic in my chest. Claire can't die without them.

"I'll have them page the daughter, they won't page anyone with the same last name." She rolled her eyes, exacerbated with the rule.

Another rule. Why do we need so many rules? It's the rules that got me into this situation in the first place. Now I was worried, momentarily, that maybe the son and the granddaughter won't pay attention to the daughter's name if they hear it announced over the public administrations system.

Within seconds, the phone rang. The unit secretary told me the son was on the phone. Oh, thank goodness he was paying attention. I picked up the phone and asked, "Are you in the waiting room?"

"Yes, I'm just down the hall." His reply was filled with questions.

"Come back to the ICU." Before I could say another word, I heard the click of the receiver in my ear.

As I dashed past the commotion, I saw the code team was still rallying around Claire's bed. The doctor had moved to the foot of the bed. The respiratory therapists were at the head of the bed, providing vital oxygen to Claire's lungs. The orderly continued circulating the blood with his strong effective CPR. My relief charge nurse was patiently waiting for another order to give more medications.

Once again, I flew out to the ICU waiting area. I looked around and saw the same people who were there the last time I was hopelessly searching. I looked down the hallway, into the small side room, and even down the back hall that leads to the stairs, still no son, no granddaughter. None of that large extended family was anywhere to be seen. *What hall did he say he was down? I don't see him in any of my halls.*

As I circled around to go back into ICU, I notice the volunteer sitting outside the ICU door. Young and innocent, she sat at the small makeshift desk to help control the visitors for the nurses. Her job was to question everyone who wants to enter the ICU and obtain permission from the nurse before letting them enter. She suddenly became one more chance of hope.

"I'm looking for family members of Claire." I describe vaguely how the son and the grand daughter look.

"If you see them, come get me in ICU 8." I instructed.

As I once again turned to leave, she looked over my shoulder and said, "There they are now."

The two of them, arm in arm, were walking hurriedly toward me. I saw fright in their faces, just as I was sure they saw in mine. I chose my words wisely as I explained to them that she had seemed to be tolerating the bi-pap fine. "I had noticed her heart rate had been slowing over the period of the last few hours. I wanted to give the bi-pap a try to see if it would work. At first she seemed to be doing fine. Shortly after we initiated the bi-pap, I noticed her heart rate dropped into the 60's. That's when I decided we needed to call the doctor to come and intubate her. The bi-pap was not going to be enough breathing support for her." I went on to say that I asked the other nurse to call the doctor while I called the respiratory therapist. "As I was bringing the module to the bed, I noticed a change in her heart rhythm, that's when I decide to call a code and get the emergency doctor to intubate her."

Both sets of eyes remained locked on my face. Every word that was exiting my mouth was being studied. I continued with my explanation of events. "We intubated her very quickly and never lost her pulse."

Just as I detected a small sigh, I had to interrupt the relief with "But, after we intubated her, her heart went into a very unstable rhythm and quickly stopped."

Once again, the fear returned to both faces simultaneously. Tears were building, now in three pair of eyes. I went on to explain that we, the code team, were doing CPR right now, trying to get the heart started again. I gave them a moment to collect their thoughts then ask the question that not many nurses will ask.

"Do you want to come in? You can be there if you want." And I waited, as they contemplated.

The son indicateded "no" just as the granddaughter nodded "yes."

"I've done it before, I want to be there," she told her father. Quickly they turned as one toward the ICU door. Dad decided, even though he didn't really want to see his mom go through this, he didn't want his daughter to witness it alone.

I led them through the door, near the bedside, but not too close. They wrapped their arms around each other and watched as the oversized orderly was compressing grandma's chest. An entire team was doing everything possible to save her life.

I left them to hold each other and moved closer to the bed. I made sure the entire code team heard me say, "The family is over there." Several eyes looked in the direction of the already grieving pair.

Families at the bedside during a code situation are not always encouraged in the ICU. For many years, we would send the family members out of the room while we, the code team, tried to bring the patient back to life. We would send them out of the room so they weren't in our way and so we didn't have to deal with them. More recently, we have started inviting the family to the room if they want to be there. This allows them to see what was being done, rather than waiting in a small room and having a stranger, who just happens to be the emergency doctor, come tell them forty five minutes later, that we did all we could but their loved one did not make it.

The code team needed to be aware that the family was watching and listening. ICU and Code Blue's are stressful situations. Some of us respond to stress in different ways. The family may interpret laughing, joking, crying, and similar responses as disrespectful. We don't want any staff members to say or do anything that will not be appropriate in this situation.

As we continued CPR, the family watched. Now they could see that we were doing everything possible. The emergency doctor walked away from the bed and toward the two hovering family members. He told them the same thing I had already explained to them. That's a good thing. They needed to hear it all again so it could sink in. Then he went back to lead the Code Blue orchestra.

Suddenly, I thought of the rest of the family. They were not here, where were they?

"Where is the rest of your family?" I asked, remembering that there were as least a dozen who were patiently taking turns visiting earlier.

"They all went to my sister's house." I could see in his facial expression that he suddenly had the same thought that I had. Maybe they should be here now.

"Do you want me to call your sister?" I inquired.

Another nod, "Yes." Very few words were coming out right now. It was all he could do to nod. The strength that he would have to use to verbalize any words was being consumed by his emotions as he watched his own mother lie in the bed, being resuscitated by a team of medical personnel. I left the two of them, once again, to call the sister. I couldn't tell her over the phone that her mother was trying to die, so I simply told her she needed to return to the hospital right away. I'm sure she could read my voice over the phone. She simply said "We're on our way," and once again I heard the click of yet another telephone receiver.

As the two stood watching and wondering, Claire's cardiologist came back into the ICU. As usual, we had called him to let him know we were coding his patient. He was not far away when he received the disturbing call, so he decided to return to the hospital. Not many doctors do that.

"It's nice to give them a personal touch," he said, referring to the family who desperately needed any touch of comfort at this time.

Well good for you! There are not too many Marcus Welby's left in this world. It's good to know that some physicians still take their oath seriously. I admire this man more today because of this one incident than any other outstanding event he has done in the fifteen years I have worked with him.

We continued trying to reverse the death that had occurred for Claire. Two doctors and myself were keeping the family informed step by step. After forty-five minutes of unsuccessful interventions, we could not get Claire's heart to beat solo again.

It's time to stop, the doctor told the family. We had done everything we could to reverse what we so desperately didn't want to happen.

The son and the granddaughter stood, latched to each other as they had been for what seemed like an eternity. Now, there was no stopping the tears. The sadness exploded, as they held tight to each other, giving and receiving support from each other. After a few moments of undisturbed grieving, the son looked at me with eyes of defeat, "What do we do now?"

Externally he was taking command of the situation. Doing what he felt he needed to do. Internally, I could see that he was in turmoil, holding back what he didn't want a room of strangers to see.

"Why don't you go out into the waiting room while we clean up, then you can come back in and see her." This would allow them some time alone to absorb what they had just experienced. The mixed up emotions were swirling through their saddened eyes. The only thing I could give them right now was a few moments of undisturbed time.

Another nod showed me that he once again agreed with my suggestion.

This time, it was their turn to use the small side room for grieving. I evacuated the others and allowed this family some quiet space to cry and hug.

We scurried to clean the area around Claire. Needle caps, medication caps, small pieces of paper littered the floor. We removed the tubes that had been inserted in desperation to keep her alive. We cleaned her face, placed a new gown on her cold body, a clean sheet on her bed, and finally placed a few chairs at the side of the bed.

After everything was clean and tidy, I once again led the family to the bedside. This time they all came in together. They crowded around the bed, they cried, and they held hands. Arrangements had to be made, people had to be called, all for this lovely lady who was vacationing with her daughter just three short weeks ago.

My shift was over; it had been for almost an hour. I stopped by the bedside to say good-bye to the family. They thanked me for all my hard work. I apologized for their loss, or maybe I was apologizing for what I was not able to do. They thanked me again.

I emptied my pockets into my locker, picked up my purse and left down the back stairs. Tears of sadness, tears of grief, tears of frustration, and probably tears of exhaustion started flowing down my cheeks. This time I wasn't content that the patient was going home to the sky. This time I wanted the patient to stay here on earth so she could vacation with her family once again.

✳ ✳ ✳

Code Blue is an alert that is announced for emergency situations—an opportunity to save lives. New, inexperienced nurses shy away and try to avoid the situation and often have tears of disappointment. More than twenty years later, older, more experienced nurses still have tears of disappointment.

Death is a common occurrence in the ICU, but it never becomes routine. Each situation is unique, each patient is unique, and each family has their own unique beliefs and needs. The nurse deals with many variations of death situations; those that come sudden and unexpected, and those that come at the end of a long, chronic illness. Even though the families have been told their loved one will die, when the time comes, it is still a shocking experience. The reality that the family member is no longer with them is often devastating.

The nurse plays an important role when supporting the family through this hard time. Physical, intellectual, and emotional support is vital for a peaceful end-of-life event. The nurse is the one at the bedside either during the code or during the last breaths of the dying patient's life. She will be the one to communicate with the family and allow them to be a part of this last event, if they choose. She will touch, hug, and provide physical presence that the family needs. It is the nurse who will answer the questions when the family asks, "What next?" and "What do we do now?" She will bring more tissues to wipe away tears. She will provide emotional support—knowing when to be close and when to keep her distance. She will be considerate of the religious and cultural needs of the family. Finally, it is the nurse who will cry with the family as they say their last good-byes, because death, though frequent, never becomes routine.

CHAPTER 5

The Gift of Life

Donating organs can save the lives of many.
Giving part of yourself can save a life.

Organ donation; many know about the little pink dot that is offered to all California drivers. That pink dot alerts others of your wishes to donate parts of your body at the time of death. Organ donation can save lives. There are many people who suffer from a variety of irreversible ailments. Heart failure, lung failure, liver failure, kidney failure, and blindness are only some inflictions that cannot be reversed and progress to the point where transplants are the only option.

Death is a natural occurrence; we will all die sooner or later. I think it is easier to deal with this unfortunate event if you believe that there is a wonderful, peaceful place where we will all go after death. I find it easier to deal with the passing of older patients, because I can rationalize that they have lived a long happy life.

But, dealing with the untimely ending of a young person's life is, of course, more difficult. They have not had a chance to do whatever it was that they were meant to do.

Finally, it is expected that old people will die, but young people are supposed to live to be old before they die. The secret to dealing with this unwanted event, time after time, is to look at the positive side. The positive outcome may be donating parts of our body that we no longer need.

There are several ways to donate after death. The first is tissue donation. This is considered at the time of *every* death in California. Tissues such as corneas, bones, skin, heart valves, and veins can be taken from patients after death and used for other living persons in need. Corneas can be transplanted to allow a blind person to see. Skin and bone can be used for grafts. Heart valves and veins can be used for various surgeries. There are many parts of the body that are simply discarded that could enhance the lives of many others in need.

Every death must be reported to the Donor Network in California. The nurse phones the Donor Network and gives the coordinator information about the deceased; the type of illness, the cause of death, any medical history, and any infections or contagious illnesses are all reported. The transplant coordinator gathers all the pertinent information and decides if the patient may be a potential tissue donor. If there is a reason why this patient is not a candidate to donate tissue—such as a contagious or infectious disease—the coordinator will release the case and nothing will be done. If, however, it is decided that the patient may be a potential tissue donor, the transplant coordinator will make a phone call to the family members and discuss this option. Tissue donation can improve the quality of life for as many as fifty to sixty individuals.

Organ donation, on the other hand, will do more than improve the quality of life. Organ donations can save lives, and may save as many as eight lives at one time. Organ donation is the giving of ones major organs; heart, lungs, kidneys, liver, and pancreas, can all be transplanted into others. Organ donation is more complicated and less common than tissue donation. Unlike tissue donation, organ donation cannot be done after the patient's heart has stopped, with very few exceptions. Organ donation is a more complicated process.

* * *

Jordan was a 32-year-old male who enjoyed riding his motor-cycle on warm sunny days. Unfortunately, Jordan was on his motorcycle one bright afternoon and the driver of another vehicle did not see him. He collided with a pickup truck and sustained massive injuries. His heart had stopped, but thanks to the quick actions of the paramedics, he was resuscitated at the scene of the accident and his heart was once again beating. His family was elated that he was alive; he had survived a horrendous accident.

Jordan was in our ICU, attached to life support machines. At the time of the cardiac arrest, he had been intubated—a tube was inserted into his lungs and attached to a ventilator. The ventilator was now breathing for Jordan and was providing oxygen to his tissues and organs in a way that he could not do for himself. IV fluids were infusing through a large vein in his neck. The bedside monitor was monitoring his blood pressure, his heart rate, and his oxygen level. There was not a mark on his body, no bruises, no abrasions, and no broken bones. He looked as if he was sleeping peacefully, but Jordan was not sleeping. He was unconscious—he was in a coma. The CT scan, previously completed in the emergency room, showed massive blood and swelling throughout his brain. It was not likely that Jordan would survive the brain damage that had occurred in the crash.

The doctors explained to his family that he had extensive brain damage and the prognosis was poor. The plan was to "wait and see," wait and see what would happened in the next few days. Usually when a patient comes into the ICU with massive brain damage, the doctors will continue to monitor, assess, and consider all options for a few days before making any final decisions. No one wants to make any quick decisions, give up too soon, or give the family any unrealistic expectations. This is the hardest thing to do—wait, wait to see if any improvement is demonstrated.

I cared for Jordan for the next few days, monitoring his vital signs and all of his bodily functions and watching his neurological status closely. His pupils were dilated and non-reactive. Normal brain function should make the pupils constrict when a flashlight is shined into them. Reflexes were absent. Jordan exhibited no movement when a painful stimulus was inflicted on his limp extremities; pain that was meant to stimulate a response. He had no blink, no gag, and no cough reflex. His body lay, flaccid, in the bed with no signs of any brain activity.

Eventually his pale, sullen face gathered fluids that caused it to swell. His arms and legs became engorged with those same stagnate bodily liquids. His lifeless body, despite the frequent baths, started to smell of decay. I cleaned and cared for Jordan, as if he was going to get up and walk out of our unit.

One day, while bathing Jordan, I noticed that someone had broken the rules of the ICU. Someone had obviously been eating at Jordan's bedside. As my charge nurse was making rounds, I brought it to her attention.

"Someone's been eating at this bedside." I reported

"How do you know?" she inquired.

"Look, there's cottage cheese in his bed." I pointed to what I had discovered. "It looks old, maybe yesterday," I continued.

The look on her face, made me explain myself further. "Look, it's grey so it probably was from yesterday or last night."

As she continued to look at me with an uncertain gaze, I started wondering what was wrong with her reaction. Why was she just starring at me with her wide-eyes? What had I done wrong? It seemed like a long time before she spoke in response to my discovery.

"Where did you find that?" She pursued.

"It was on his sheet, next to his head, when I rolled him over," I explained.

As she moved to the head of the bed, she reached for a cotton-tipped swab from the bedside table. With that swab, she removed more of what I thought was old cottage cheese from Jordan's ear. She needed to say nothing to explain how she found more of what I thought was cottage cheese in Jordan's ear. Her look alone, told me what I didn't want to know. What I had found on his sheet, and what she had just swabbed from his ear, was not evidence that someone had broken the no eating rule. It was evidence that Jordan's brain was so swollen, that it could no longer remain confined to his skull, it was leaking out through whatever orifice it could escape.

I will never forget that day; I cleaned Jordan's face, mouth, nose, and ears every time I was at his bedside. I didn't want his family to experience what I had just experienced for the first time. I didn't want his family to live through the devastation that I had just lived through. They were grieving for their young son; they didn't need to see the physical effects of Jordan's head injury.

His family sat attentively at the bedside almost around the clock. His mother, father, aunts, uncles, cousins, and even friends who said they were cousins if necessary to gain access through the "immediate family only" visiting policy. Jordan required basic care, bathing, turning, and monitoring. But his family required more challenging care. It was the nurses who had to care for the grieving family members. It was the nurses who had to prepare the family for the eventual outcome. It was the nurses who had to sit and talk and listen to the stories of how Jordan was the best son, the best cousin, and the best friend. And it was the nurses who had to answer all the questions and explain why Jordan looked so good, but wasn't. Caring for the needs of the family quickly became more difficult and complicated than caring for Jordan.

* * *

Brain death—terminology used when the brain is no longer functioning—is the total and irreversible loss of all brain activity. How can a person look so alive, but be brain dead? Unlike cardiac death, brain death does not always result in immediate cessation of life, as we know it. Brain death occurs when the brain stops functioning. Death has occurred, but if the heart is revived and oxygenated, it will continue to beat automatically. The heart is an automatic muscle, as long as it has oxygen, the heart muscle will continue to contract and the heart will beat. In order to provide the needed oxygen to the heart, the patient must be breathing. If the patient cannot breathe on his own, we can put a tube in his lungs and breathe for him with a ventilator. As long as the ventilator is providing oxygen to the heart, the heart will continue to pump. But that doesn't mean the brain is working, and that doesn't mean the patient is alive, he is technically dead.

There are two types of death, cardiac death and brain death. Cardiac death occurs when the heart stops. When the heart stops, blood is no longer circulated to the body and the vital organs stop working. Without an adequate blood supply, the organs do not receive the oxygen needed to function. Cardiac death results in loss of circulation and loss of life. It is obvious when a patient has suffered from a cardiac death; there is no pulse and no respirations.

It is less obvious when a patient has suffered from brain death. Because these patients are often on life support, a ventilator to breathe for them, and the oxygenation allows for the automaticity of the heart to continue to beat, it appears that they are alive. But they are not.

When the patient's condition is grave and there seems to be almost no neurological response, the nurse is required to contact the Donor Network. Jordan's condition was easily identified as a potential donor. His age and his lack of brain responses were red flags for organ donation possibilities. The nurse provides information to the transplant coordinator; the network staff will discuss the case and decide if there is potential for donation. The patient information is entered into the database for follow-up monitoring. If the patient has not been determined to be brain dead, the transplant coordinator will provide a contact number and ask the nurse to phone back if anything changes, or if the patient's condition deteriorates to brain death.

If a patient has already been pronounced brain dead, the call to the Donor Network becomes more urgent. At this time, the nurse, the physician, and the medical team may discuss donation options with the family. Many nurses may not feel comfortable discussing donation with the family, if so, the network will send a transplant coordinator to the hospital to provide the support and information to the family in order to help them make a comfortable decision.

The nurse is also not required to ask permission from the doctor to contact the Donor Network. She is not giving away any organs, she is not changing the care of the patient, and she is not making the official determination that the patient will or will not survive; she is simply alerting the Donor Network of a potential candidate. The transplant coordinator will maintain the information and respond when notified of any change by the staff.

One morning I was caring for a patient in this condition, and when the physician was making rounds, the coordinator phoned for an update. When he found out that the Donor Network was asking about his patient, he almost had a stroke of his own. He was angry that the nurses had contacted the network in the first place. I explained to him that we are required by law to inform the Network of all patients who may have a potential for neurological death, and that it was not required for the physician to provide consent for this process to be initiated. That physician was not happy, but we stood up to what we knew was right. The doctor does not determine when the Donor Network is contacted, the nurse does. And if the doctor doesn't want us to call, we do it anyway.

* * *

It was soon evident that Jordan was not going to survive. The brain tissue that was leaking from his ears, along with the continued lack of reflexes, provided me with what I needed to initiate the next step. While I continued to care for Jordan and his family, as I would any other patient, I initiated the organ donation process. I made the initial call and informed the transplant coordinator that I was caring for a young thirty-two-year-old male who had no medical history, no medical problems. I reported Jordan's current condition and my assessment of his lack of responses. The transplant coordinator collected all of the pertinent data, including age, height, weight, blood type and much more. Then I was told that they would keep in touch and I was to inform any other nurse caring for Jordan to call the network if any changes occurred. Jordan was now in the system and would be followed until the appropriate time arrived.

On the third day, the waiting was over. The test results showed that there were no brain waves, no brain activity. The neurologist came in early in the morning to make his final assessment. Because the mother was not present at the bedside, he arranged for a family conference to take place at noon. The family would gather all key members and meet with the doctor. The case manager, the one who oversees the progression of the patient's care and discharge needs, and the chaplain would join us for the conference. I called the Donor Network to tell them of the events of the day. Jordan had been pronounced dead, and we would be meeting with the family at noon.

Leslie, the coordinator from the Donor Network arrived at the hospital by ten o'clock that morning. She reviewed the chart, made several phone calls, and decided Jordan had a lot to offer. His previous health would allow him to donate multiple organs. Leslie worked diligently all morning checking, calling, and providing suggestions for maintaining adequate oxygen to all of Jordan's organs. Now we just had to wait for noon.

The doctor met with the entire family, as promised. He gently explained that Jordan's brain was no longer functioning and he was dead. Despite the fact that Jordan's chest continued to raise each time the ventilator pushed air into his lungs, and despite the fact that Jordan's heart continued to pump blood to his entire body, he was dead. The family was told that they could spend some time with Jordan, then the ventilator would be removed and they could make funeral arrangements.

The doctor left the family in the conference room, to gather their thoughts, and returned to the ICU. "I've told the family. Give them some time then we will turn off the ventilator." I informed him that Leslie, the transplant coordinator, was looking into the possibility of recovering organs. The doctor didn't need to be involved in this process. He only asked that we inform him when the process was complete.

The family came to the bedside, cried and mourned for the loss of their young family member. Each of them was given time to say their good-byes in whatever way they needed. We allowed them as much time as they needed. At one point, the parents had retreated back to the private conference room. They were involved in their own conversations and planning.

Leslie, after asking permission to enter, joined them for some conversation. Leslie, because of her additional training, was the one who approached the family with the idea of donating Jordan's organs. She sat with them for an extended amount of time. She explained the entire process. She answered all of their questions. "Donating organs," she explained, "is a way for your son to live on. The death of your son could save the life of several other people." After some private discussion, Jordan's parents told Leslie that they had decided to give life to others by giving whatever organs and tissues could be of use.

As of that moment, the transplant coordinator assumed management of the patient. The patient was officially pronounced dead earlier that morning, and the Donor Network would manage the care and pay the costs while waiting for the process to be finalized. There would be no costs of organ donation to the family. We ordered lab work to check electrolytes, and blood types among other things. We ordered x-rays and echocardiogram to check the status of the lungs and the heart. We did an ultrasound to confirm the health of the kidneys. I worked closely with Leslie, giving fluids, monitoring intake and output, maintaining adequate perfusion to all organs, while the workers on the other side of the phone were searching for recipients who would match with Jordan's blood type and organ size.

Six hours later, we took Jordan to the operating room, just as if he were going for a routine surgery. The operating room suite was set up and the staff was ready. There were several teams waiting to surgically remove the gifts that Jordan was about to give. The teams would remove the organs that they would transport to their facilities and implant into an awaiting recipient. The heart, lungs, and one kidney would be transported by limousine to a local teaching hospital. The liver and pancreas were going by helicopter to a second location. The other kidney was going to yet a third location hundreds of miles away. The organs were removed one by one, the heart last so it could continue to pump oxygen to the others until they were gently taken away. After the vital organs were removed, the tissue removal was done in less urgent manner. Both of Jordan's corneas were sent to a different location allowing two different people to have the gift of sight. A variety of other tissues were recovered for use in future surgeries.

Because of the selfless act of Jordan's parents, five lives were saved, two others regained sight, and fifty to sixty others would benefit from his tissues. Jordan lost his life in a traumatic accident, but the outcome was positive for many others.

* * *

Sometimes there are cultural and religious beliefs that interfere with the willingness to donate tissues and organs. But the idea must be presented to everyone if the situation is right. For many of us, who do not have cultural or religious beliefs that will hinder our willingness, we should all consider giving life at the time of our death. The first step to become an organ donor is to register online with the Donor Networks or with the Department of Motor Vehicles when you renew your driver's license. Many states have passed legislation regarding "first person consent" which says that only the donor must provide consent. Family cannot override this decision. But, in order to provide peace at the time of our death, we must also talk to the members of our family about donating whatever organs and body parts can be used to promote life in another. We must let our family know if we want our tissues and organs donated, and ask them if they want theirs donated. Ask your children, ask your parents, and communicate with each other so in the end, it will be easier to make the right decision and do the right thing.

✳ ✳ ✳

My son was about eleven when we had the discussion about organ donation. I was discussing this, once again, with my husband. My son entered the room and joined the conversation. I explained the process to him. When a patient's brain is no longer functioning, they are considered dead even though the heart is beating and the rest of the body seems to be alive. I asked him, if he was ever in an accident and he was brain dead, would he want me to donate his heart and lungs and kidneys to another person who could use them.

He thought about my request for a minute. I could see he was contemplating his answer. He needed to clarify some facts before he could provide the answer for which I waiting.

"My heart is working?" he asked.

"Yes," I responded.

"My lungs are working?" he continued.

"Yes, with a machine," I clarified.

"Everything is working except my brain?" he said, this time with a puzzled look in his eyes.

"Yes," with a nod of my head, I confirmed all of his thoughts. "That's why you would be considered dead. Your brain is no longer working." With this, I thought I had fully explained the random scenario that had initiated this conversation.

"No, I'd want a brain transplant," he said adamantly.

Since brain transplants are not an option, I had to further explain the only alternative in that situation would be to donate his organs rather than receive someone else's brain. We joked about what it would be like if I donated my brain to him, or he donated his to me; a boy with a mom's thought processes, or a mom with a young boy's thoughts. We wondered how that would be. And we laughed about a few oddball scenarios. In the end, he agreed, and provided me with the support that I could gift his organs to another if the time ever comes. So I, just like Jordan's parents, will give the gift of life if I should ever be faced with the decision.

To Care … But Not Too Much

When working in the ICU, the nurse has many opportunities to care for patients over a long period of time. Sometimes she will become very involved with the patient, caring for the same patient day after day, developing a relationship with the patient and the family, as she provides compassionate care for that individual human being.

Sometimes that same nurse will need to distance herself from her patient. Not because the nurse doesn't want to be involved, but because it hurts to be involved. When caring for critically ill patients, it hurts to live through the suffering, and the deaths, day after day. So, sometimes she must keep her distance, in order to keep her sanity.

But, a good nurse needs to know how to keep her distance, for her own sanity, while maintaining a comforting relationship with the patient and the family. The nurse must not be cold and uncaring, but provide the supportive care needed while allowing herself opportunities to step away when needed.

The patient and the family need support. They need to know the nurse cares, and they need to know that she will be there when necessary. We need to stay close when we can, keep our distance when we need to, but never stop caring. That's why we are in the nursing profession.

CHAPTER 6

What About Me?

When the nurse becomes the patient. What can be
learned from that experience?

What happens when a nurse gets sick? What happens when one of the family members of the nurse gets sick? What happens when the friend of a nurse gets sick, and what if that friend just happens to be a nurse too? Some say the worse patient is a doctor, and some say the worse patient is the wife of a doctor. I disagree; I think the worse patient is the nurse, who just happens to have a lot of friends who are nurses. When a doctor is admitted to the hospital, his doctor friends don't usually come, ask questions and tell the nurse what to do, they usually give him his privacy and step aside. When a doctor's wife is admitted, the doctor himself will be the one with all the questions and demands for the nurse, one additional person asking questions and telling the nurse what to do. But, when a nurse is admitted, not only is she asking questions and telling her nurse what to do, but also all of her nurse friends are there, making sure that everything is right. All the nurse friends come at different times of the day, because nurses work different shifts throughout the day. All those friends, nurses with variable background and knowledge, will ask the same questions and request a variety of tasks to be done. Those nurses are the ones who are always caring for others when they are sick. Those nurses are the ones who have been challenged daily to be a patient advocate. When one of their own is down, sick in the hospital, all of the nurse friends now become her advocates, whether she needs them or not.

Nurses react to illness in several ways. When the nurse acquires a minor ailment, like a headache, that doesn't go away quickly with the appropriate over-the-counter medications, she may start thinking; *maybe I have an intra-cerebral hemorrhage.* The nurse contemplates small pox, shingles, and allergic reaction all before the simple heat rash is considered. A cough is pneumonia. Leg pain must be a blood clot. Heavy menstrual cycles are hemorrhages. Indigestion is a heart attack. Why is this? Perhaps because the nurse has witnessed many possible illnesses that start out as simple colds, or untreated headaches, that quickly turn into disasters. Maybe the ICU nurse sees the sickest patients and correlates all illnesses with the worst of the worst. We think this, but we don't do anything about it. We imagine that we have the worst of the worse, but we don't do anything; we don't have time to be sick. The headache, the heart attack, the hemorrhages are all ignored until the symptoms are so severe they cannot be ignored any longer.

Even though the threat of contracting a disastrous illness may cross the nurse's mind, she still doesn't stop to take care of herself when she is sick. Nurses are too busy taking care of others to stop and take care of themselves. When a nurse gets sick, she still gets up to care for the kids, she still makes her husband dinner, and she still makes sure the laundry is done, like most moms and wives. And, the nurse still goes to work because she knows if she doesn't, no one else will. She must go to work to care for those more acutely sick patients. No one will come in on their day off. No one will come in because they are exhausted from their own shifts worked. The nurse works hard, so when she has a day off, she doesn't even want to think about working for anyone else. But on the other hand, when the sick nurse reports to duty, she is then contaminating the workforce with whatever virus she has, and the other nurses will soon be carrying it too. This becomes a vicious cycle of the sick getting the others sick, and then eventually no one is available to care for the acutely ill. Nurses need to learn to take care of themselves. Rest, stay home and think about others *after* thinking of themselves.

* * *

Many nurses don't take care of themselves. They know they need to address an illness but they don't want to know the implications. Or perhaps, they do know the implications and just don't want to admit it. For example, I rarely experience indigestion, but one night I woke up with heartburn. Because this is rare for me, I wasn't sure what I should do. Rather than getting out of bed and taking a chewable antacid, I lay there contemplating whether I was having a heart attack. The pressure in my chest was minor at first. I know that heart attacks don't always come on with severe pain. I was sure, for one minute, that it was just indigestion. I decided to wait a few minutes more to see if it would go away. As I waited, the fact that my family history is riddled with heart disease came to mind. But again, I reassured myself that it must have been something that I ate.

It must have been at least five minutes that I lay awake. The pressure started getting worse. It wasn't going away. Then I started making a plan. *What will I do if it keeps getting worse? What if it doesn't go away?* But, did I get out of my warm comfortable bed to get one of those fruit-flavored chewables? No, I started planning my emergency room visit. *Should I wake my husband? Should I call 911? Or should I get dressed first?* No way was I going to wear my pajamas, especially since I know everyone in the emergency room who would be caring for me. Never go to the emergency in your pajamas. I remembered one of the emergency room nurses commenting that the staff thinks that it's absurd when patients come in their pajamas.

Another ten minutes passed slowly. I am not one to wake up in the middle of the night. If I wake up, it doesn't take long to go immediately back to sleep. Now I was getting annoyed. How dare this discomfort interrupt my precious sleep. Even though the pressure in my chest continued, I started doubting myself. *I might be having a heart attack. But what if I'm not? What if I get to the emergency room and the pain suddenly goes away. What if I get there and they find my EKG is normal? What if I embarrass myself by calling 911 and nothing is wrong? What if I have my husband drive me and I have a sudden death in the car on the way.* I decided to wait, wait until the pain is really bad, not just annoying. I'd wait until I was sure I was having a heart attack before I would go to the emergency room in the middle of the night, despite the fact that we, healthcare providers, repeatedly tell the public, not to delay care, especially if they think they may be having a heart attack. I've worked a few shifts in the emergency room and I know there are a lot of people who go there for no good reason. I was not going to be one of them. So, I waited a few more minutes, and the indigestion went away. I drifted off to sleep, and I didn't die in my sleep from a heart attack.

Nurses, especially ICU nurses, don't want to think that they could be sick or injured. ICU nurses experience multiple illnesses daily, with our patients that do not always end up with the positive outcomes we hope for.

* * *

Another example of how I chose to ignore a potential illness occurred many years ago, when I took my son ice-skating for his tenth birthday. I hadn't been ice-skating for several years before that skating party. I, of course, had to go out on the ice and prove that I was still the ice skater that I had once been. As I was showing those young boys how a mom could skate, I took a fall. One foot flew forward to the right and one foot flew forward to the left. My tailbone was the first to hit the rock hard ice, followed quickly by the back of my head. Crack—I heard my skull meet the ice. I quickly looked around to see how many people had just witnessed me making a fool of myself. No one was watching, at least no one continued to stare once I composed myself enough to look around. If anyone had seen the fall, they had tactfully looked away before I could see them gawking at my embarrassing event. I slowly picked myself up off the ice, and found my way to the outlet of the floor while holding the life-saving railing. I gently walked those ice skates on the carpet to the ladies room where I massaged the knot that immediately started growing on the back of my head. I took off those skates and replaced them with my comfortable sneakers, assured that I could maintain an upright position with those. I managed to keep my cool through the remainder of the birthday party. Acetaminophen alleviated the headache that quickly overtook my entire skull. The remainder of the evening was uneventful and the party was a success despite the large egg on the back of my head.

The next morning, I awoke spinning. As I turned to get out of bed, I felt like I was on the ceiling fan. Boy was I dizzy. I lay back in bed, waited a few minutes then rolled off the side. Immediately I ran to the bathroom to vomit. I could hardly stand. I needed to hold onto the wall to keep from stumbling. I returned to bed and tried not to move. Each time I moved, I threw up. Each time I opened my eyes I found myself spinning endlessly. There was no way I was getting out of that bed. Some kind of flu bug, boy this one knocked me this time.

My husband got the boys off to school and I was content to stay in bed. Because I vomited every time I moved, I chose not to move. This too would pass, as long as I didn't move, I'd be fine. Midmorning the phone rang. I had to debate whether I could move slowly enough to reach it without heaving into the wastebasket that was left by my bed. I managed to reach the phone and heard the voice of my good friend. Julie missed me at work that day and was wondering what was wrong. I never missed a day of work; it was not like me to call in sick. I explained to her what I was suffering through.

"This is sure a bad flu," I whined.

"Are you kidding me!" was her immediate response.

"What?" Why was she yelling at me when I was so sick?

"Didn't you tell me that you just cracked your skull on the ice yesterday? Don't you think this could be related? Did you ever think that you might have an intracranial hemorrhage?"

Wow, too many questions. But boy did she shake some sense into me. She was right, head injury followed by abnormal neurological signs. Dizziness, nausea, vomiting are all signs of neurological changes. Now I was sure I had an intracranial hemorrhage. *Oh no, who was going to raise my boys?* I had gone from minimizing this event as the flu to maximizing the event as preceding my death with one short phone call from my best friend, who just happened to be a nurse, too.

My next call was to my husband. By now I was in tears, scared because I was exhibiting neurological changes related to increased intracranial pressure. Scared that I was going to have my head shaved for surgery. I had already convinced myself that the surgeon would need to evacuate the hematoma that was putting pressure on my brain and causing those neurological changes. I was scared that if I didn't get to the hospital soon, I would probably require long-term rehab. Who would take care of my family? On the other hand, the entire time I was telling my husband that I needed to go the hospital, I was telling myself that I really didn't want to do this. It was only because Julie was making me. I was sure it was nothing. Julie was trying to convince me that I could truly be in trouble, while I was trying to convince myself that it was truly nothing. My husband left his job and came home to find me in emotional turmoil. It was better to be safe than sorry. He convinced me to listen to my friend and get checked by a doctor. As I walked to the car, holding onto the walls along the way, I tried not to throw up.

Any time a fellow nurse enters the emergency room as a patient, looking like she just got out of bed and not caring, the staff knows something is not right. That morning, I didn't care who looked at my dried-on make-up, who saw my uncombed hair, or who smelled my morning breath. As I was trying hard not to vomit on their paperwork, my husband explained to the triage nurse that I had taken a hard fall on the ice yesterday and today had neurological symptoms of dizziness and vomiting. She agreed with my good friend, that it was too much of a coincidence to ignore.

As with all employees, they sent me into a room immediately, no waiting. I spent the next few hours waiting, being examined, waiting, being sent to the CT scanner, and waiting for the doctor to come back and tell me I had labrynthitis, a minor ailment of the inner ear that causes dizziness and motion sickness-type symptoms. After I was sent home, I spent the next few hours complaining that my good friend made me go to the emergency room and all those people saw me looking crappy. But, who would have known? I could have had major problems related to that fall on the ice. It's a good thing that we nurses have nurse friends to take care of us, because we certainly don't take care of ourselves.

* * *

We nurses take care of each other. We look out for each other, like we take care of our patients. But do we take care of everyone the same? The nurse cares for those who cannot care for themselves. We provide for every aspect of their needs when they are experiencing major illness and dying. How do we react to minor illnesses? How are we with our family members? Do we give them the same sympathy and concern that we give our critically ill patients? Another dilemma for contemplation.

My husband often complains that he gets no sympathy from me. He wonders how I can care so much for those patients in the hospital, but care so little for him when he is sick? My husband is never sick, well almost never. His idea of sick is a headache, a cold, a muscle ache, and occasionally, the flu. Those are not major illnesses. Those are daily events that everyone must simply deal with and overcome. The average nurse, and wife, does not even slow down when she has a headache. The average nurse just keeps on going through that cold and doesn't even think of it as a sickness. And the average nurse suffers daily with muscle aches. Our backs are taxed and abused on a daily basis and we just keep on going.

My husband, however, must have thought that if he married a nurse, I would become his handmaiden and take care of him when he had the least little illness. "Get over it," is my response. No whining allowed in my house; there is absolutely no tolerance for complaining about minor ailments. "You think you are sick, you should see the patients I take care of." After a few years, my husband learned that in order to get any sympathy from me, when he is sick, he will have to have a predetermined number of tubes inserted in various areas of his body. Now, after many years of marriage, he has learned that my sympathy is used up at work for those who can't care for themselves. A minor ailment is nothing to complain about. I do make sure my family is cared for when ill, as all mothers do, but not to the level that was expected as a newlywed. Find yourself a life-threatening illness, have a variety of physicians insert tubes into several of your orifices, and you will gain my sympathy. As long as you are healthy and able to care for yourself, my skills and sympathy are better used elsewhere.

Skills, sympathy and compassion are used daily in nursing. It's not until a nurse becomes a patient that she realizes how important these traits are. When that same nurse who has imagined many times that she is terminally ill with that headache or that indigestion, but doesn't do anything except take an over the counter medication, lands in the hospital bed herself, she learns very quickly how important compassion is. When hospitalized, that nurse will do anything not to be a burden to the other nurses. She doesn't want the other nurses to spend their precious time helping her when there are probably many more patients that deserve the time. She doesn't want the other nurses to have to do things for her that she can do for herself. And, she doesn't even want to go to the hospital in the first place. She knows that sick people go there and she doesn't have time to be sick.

* * *

A few years ago, I became a patient at the same hospital where I worked. That was an experience I will never forget. It started with some vague abdominal pain. Left upper quadrant pain that seemed to become sharp stabbing pains when I would take a deep breath. I went to see my doctor who prescribed some antispasmodic medications.

"Come back if this doesn't help." That's always what they say when they don't know what they are dealing with.

I tried the medications, but within a week I was back in the office. This time I was telling my doctor "It feels like I have a tear in my diaphragm." As if I would know what a torn diaphragm felt like, but it was what I imagined it would feel like. Whenever I took a deep breath, whenever I laughed, and God forbid I should hiccough, the pain was excruciating. The pain was not getting better with the medication, it was getting worse. Something was wrong. And now I was in his office, crying in pain

What's good for a crying woman with abdominal pain in the doctor's office? An intramuscular injection of pain medication. But that didn't work. The shot helped the pain, but I wasn't satisfied. Why was I having pain? I knew pain is a symptom of something, and something was wrong. This time I knew that whatever was wrong was not going away with over-the-counter medications and patience.

My doctor sent me, the following day, to a gastroenterologist. Since I had called my mother the previous day to pick me up from the doctor's office—after the pain medication—there was no way she was going to let me go alone to the next doctor's appointment. So, as we all need to do, we let our mothers help us when they feel they need to. Well, little did I know just how much I was going to need my mother on that day.

After the specialist examined me, he excused himself from the room. "Get dressed, I'll be right back." They all say that. I expected him to come back in, give me his opinion, and give me a prescription and send me home.

This time, it wasn't as I expected. When the specialist reentered the examination room, he told me he wanted to make a call, and he wanted me to hear the conversation. He dialed the phone in the room and immediately made arrangements for my admission to the hospital.

"I'm not sure what's going on, but I want to do some tests," is all that he would say. At that time, I didn't realized how concerned he was by the look in his eyes. Later, he would confess to me his true concerns.

I tried to negotiate with him. "Can I go do a few things? I need to run to the mall and purchase a birthday present for my son to take to the party this weekend?"

"No."

"Let me go put a load of clothes in the washer, and do some grocery shopping for the family so they will have food for the weekend."

"No."

"Can I at least go home and take a shower and shave my legs."

"No, absolutely not. Your mother will drive you directly to the hospital, now." He remained adamant about no delays.

Now I was worried. I had never been admitted to the hospital before, except for childbirth. I had things to do. This was a long weekend, and the boys had places to be. But that doctor was not budging. I was to go directly to the hospital, no detours, and no delays. My mother obeyed the doctor and did exactly what she was told. I guess she doesn't know that ICU nurses don't always listen to the doctors. But, she drove me directly to the hospital.

I entered my own hospital, like so many others do and I walked to the admitting department. I told the admitting clerk who I was and who had sent me. She already had the information in front of her. She would expedite my admission as quickly as possible. While I was waiting, my good friend Julie came to my rescue. She was there in the admitting department to make sure that I would be admitted to a room on "her floor." She was a manager of the 7th floor and she wanted me in that unit where she could be my advocate, as we all do for each other.

I had lab tests, chest x-ray, and a lung scan. There was an accumulation of fluid around the lung. The nuclear medicine technician, doing the lung scan, was very polite; she did a good job at maintaining my dignity, knowing that we were both employees. She maintained her professional attitude, while reassuring me through my anxious thoughts.

My experience in the CT scanner was not as enjoyable. The x-ray technician performed the CT scan in a short time. He, however, was not as dignified as the nuclear medicine technician. As I was moving off the table, I did what we all do. I asked for the results. I figured since I was a nurse, and he knew it, he might divulge a little information. After all, when I bring my patients into his CT scanner, he always tells me what he sees. But, that is an unofficial opinion of the technician, and we always wait for the radiologist to provide us with an official result of all tests.

Well, little did I know this technician was about to let me know how smart he thought he was. He was going to tell me exactly what he saw in the scan. His first response to my inquiry was some exploration of his own.

"You haven't been very hungry lately, have you?" he inquired.

The pain hadn't really affected my appetite. I assured him of that.

"Pain was your only symptom?" he asked.

"Yes," I assured him. Followed by the ultimate question "Why, what did you see?"

I had no idea what I was about to hear. The technician told me that he had seen a huge tumor. He also told me that the tumor was so big that it was pushing my stomach to one side, and it was also pushing my kidney out of the way as well. I heard nothing else after that. He pushed the gurney I was on all the way to my newly assigned room. He talked the entire time it took to ride the elevator up seven floors, journey to the end of the hall, and assist me to my waiting hospital bed. But after I heard "big tumor," I heard nothing else of his long lengthy conversation.

I positioned myself in my bed so I wouldn't have to look at him as he left the room. I didn't want to see the person who had just delivered the information that he had shared with me.

"Take care," he said, as he strolled lightheartedly down the hall.

Take care. How could I take care? I have cancer throughout my entire abdomen, a huge tumor that was displacing all of my internal organs. Take care? After what he had told me, he simply said, "take care."

It's hard to explain my feelings at that moment. I felt disbelief that this was really happening. *I'm the nurse; I'm the one who takes care of the sick, not the one who gets sick.* I felt doubt that he really knew what he saw. *Maybe he just thinks he knows what he was looking at, maybe he really didn't see a huge tumor.* I felt fright, I was afraid of what was going to happen next. I was afraid that I had cancer and I was going to die. I was afraid of what would happen to my family. Most of all, I felt anger, that he had told me what he saw. Didn't he know when I asked he should have denied that he saw anything? He should have said he would have to wait for the radiologist to read the film. Even if he did see something, he shouldn't have told me. That technician had no business telling me what he saw in those films. That technician caused me an entire night of grief. I lay in that bed, worrying until morning, when the doctor came and told me the official results of the scan.

I had a mass on my spleen. No one was sure what it was, but it needed to be removed. I was scheduled for surgery a few days later. My surgeon insisted on waiting a few days in order to allow the pneumonia vaccine some time to work. Pneumonia vaccine, the vaccine that is given to those who lose a spleen in order to boost immunity, and help prevent pneumonia, was essential now. While waiting in that hospital bed, I started preparing my family for the worse. I made sure my family knew that the spleen is an incredibly vascular organ. And if there was more bleeding than was expected, the surgeon may put me in ICU after the surgery.

"Don't be alarmed if he tells you I am in the ICU." I assured them "That will be just a precaution." I wanted them to be prepared and not to worry. After all, I was worrying enough for all of us.

The surgery went well; the doctor removed a benign cyst that was encapsulating my spleen along with my entire spleen, and I returned to the same room I was in previously for an uneventful recuperation. My best friend, the nurse manager, made sure all my needs were met. The nurses were all very attentive and professional. One of the most uncomfortable experiences was the naso-gastric tube—the tube that entered through my nose and traveled down to my stomach. It kept my stomach empty. The diameter of the tube was about one centimeter—less than one-half inch. But it felt like a garden hose had been passed into my stomach. My throat was constantly dry and the pain in my nose and throat was exaggerated every time anyone even thought of touching that tube.

As I lay in bed complaining about that small naso-gastric tube, I thought about all of my ICU patients who had these tubes. Now I realized the agony they go through. Many of my ICU patients have endotracheal tubes as well. The endotracheal tubes are twice as big as the one I had, and go directly into the lungs, causing coughing and choking, in addition to pain, when moved or touched. I had a naso-gastric tube only. My ICU patients have a naso-gastric tube and an endotracheal tube, one going through the nose into the stomach and another going through the mouth into the lungs. I developed a new understanding of what my patients' experience with annoying tubes.

I also developed a new understanding of how important the little things are when being a patient. One morning while I was administering my own sponge bath, one of my co-workers came to see me on her morning break. I'm not a modest person, so I invited her in as I completed my task. I had washed my face and my armpits and was going to call it quits. I was feeling refreshed by the warm water and cloth in the appropriate places. As I pushed the basin of water away, Carol asked me if I wanted her to wash my back.

"No thanks, I'm fine," I assured her.

That was not fine for her. "Let me sponge your back." This time she "asked" with a little more emphasis.

"No really, it's O.K." I didn't want her to spend her break time caring for me.

Now she was insisting. Since I had denied her request, it was now a *demand.* She picked up the cloth, soaked it with warm water, squeezed to prevent dripping on the linens, and proceeded to gently sponge my back. As she stroked up and down my bare back, I could feel the tension leaving my body. The combination of the warm water and gentle massage was better medicine than any pain reliever could have been. This simple task of sponging my back meant so much to me. One would never think that simple tasks could be so comforting. This event also provided me with a new understanding of the small touches.

✳ ✳ ✳

Today, when caring for my patients, I am more sympathetic to their needs. I understand the discomfort they are experiencing with the unwanted tubes. And, I always insist on sponging the backs of those who are able to provide their own personal care. Even if the patient insists that it is not needed, I find a way to convince them, just as Carol convinced me. I remember how good it felt, and I want my patients to remember, too. For those patients who cannot provide their own care, I always provide a comforting bath for them. In between baths, usually done daily, I provide additional skin care and massage with lotion, along with fresh linens. It's easy to provide small touches of care that result in an unbelievable amount of comfort.

All nurses should become a patient at some point in their career. This would allow each individual to experience the bad along with the good. They will realize how it feels to have tubes in every orifice; yet how relaxing a back rub feels.

As a patient, the nurse sees things from the other side of the bed. Being a patient allows the nurse to experience what it feels like when it takes too long to answer a call light. Being a patient allows the nurse to experience the time lag after asking for pain medications. And, being a patient allows the nurse to provide better care for her patients for the rest of her career.

CHAPTER 7

Super Size Me

*What changes our attitude about those who are
morbidly obese and too big to fit in the bed?*

Obesity is the medical term used to describe an overweight person. When a person is more than twenty percent over the ideal body weight, they are technically considered obese. Obesity in America is everywhere, some say as many as one-third of the American population is obese. We simply have to look around to see many people who are obese. Morbidly obese is a term used to describe a patient who is so overweight, usually one-hundred pounds over the ideal body weight, which results in health problems and an increased risk of death. Morbidly obese people endure discrimination every day. Whether we admit it or not, many of us have looked at "fat" people in a discriminatory way. Many think they are lazy slobs who don't care about themselves. Many of us have looked at fat people in scooters and thought to ourselves, *if they would just lose a few pounds, they could walk and not need that scooter.* Many of us have seen overweight people at buffet restaurants and thought, *boy are they getting their moneys worth.* But, how many of us personally know one of those overly large people. How many of us know what is deep inside each of those huge bodies. I had many of these same thoughts and feelings until I met some morbidly obese patients in my ICU.

* * *

Peter came to our hospital one calm autumn evening. He was brought to the emergency room like many other patients, by ambulance. The emergency medical technicians (EMT's) had radioed ahead and alerted the department that they were bringing "a rather obese gentleman, complaining of hip pain." No other complaints were relayed through the radio. The first thoughts of the nurses were, *why would a patient need to come by ambulance when his only complaint was a sore hip? Must be a fracture.*

As the bay doors opened to allow the gurney to enter, the staff understood why the ambulance was used. Instead of the two-person crew who usually accompany ambulance patients, Peter had a team of fire fighters with him. As the four strapping men pushed the gurney into the cubical, the second gurney was briskly whisked out of the way. A flurry of nurses, doctors, and technicians gathered around the gurney to assure prompt response to what they were alerted to prior to arrival. During transport, in the ambulance, the patient's seemingly stable condition deteriorated. Now, the hip pain was moved down on the list of priorities as the staff gathered information.

They were quick to assess the needs of this newly arrived patient. Technicians ran from room to room finding an extra large blood pressure cuff to monitor vital signs, a bed sheet to cover his large body in order to provide some privacy, and repositioned the equipment in the room to make space for the needed care. Nurses worked quickly to start IV's, draw blood specimens, and support the physician.

All as the physician positioned himself at the head of the bed to gather his own data while assessing the patient and pulling together the data provided him by his team members. It didn't take long for the emergency room doctor to start formulating a plan.

Peter's blood pressure was 80/50, his heart rate was 124 beats per minute, and his temperature was 102 degrees. Peter had some kind of infection that was causing his body to go into shock. Infection that gets into the blood stream and affects the entire body systems is called sepsis. Peter was obviously septic and he needed immediate treatment or he could die.

IV fluids were poured into Peter's weak body, cultures were sent to the lab, and antibiotics were started, all while trying to determine the site of the infections. Untreated pneumonia can sometimes result in sepsis, so the doctor ordered a chest x-ray.

"X-ray that sore hip while you're at it." It seemed, perhaps, he thought the hip pain was unrelated to the other more alarming issues he had discovered.

As the portable x-ray machine rolled into the cubical, the team worked to position Peter. As they pushed and pulled him from side to side, a new discovery proved to provide vital information about the cause of the pain, the temperature, and the septic shock.

The doctor was quickly summoned back to the cubical. Several staff members rolled Peter to the side to allow complete visibility. A wound appeared from beneath the folds of excessive weight. Pressure of his oversized body had caused a wound that had been hidden beneath the areas of neglect.

Initially the wound looked insignificantly small on the side of this large buttock, but as the nurse placed her average size hand next to this newly discovered obligation, it quickly become apparent that the small wound was half again the width of her hand. Against the background of the endless skin it looked small, but next to the reality of real size comparison the significance became more apparent. The glossy scarlet red sphere was encircled by the roughness of the darkened gray border. The redness faded into the surrounding tissues as if to disappear into nowhere. It was now obvious that the hip pain was most likely caused by this pressure ulcer that had been growing for an unknown amount of time.

The wound was cultured, cleaned and covered as ordered by the physician. The x-ray was done just to make sure that the initial conclusion, that this was the cause of the pain, was not incorrect. We would check for any broken bones, just in case.

The distraction of the wound was short lived when the blood pressure was not responding to fluids. Vasopressors, medications to support the blood pressure, were started. Levophed drip would help lift the blood pressure while the fluids had a chance to fill the most likely dilated vasculature. The team continued to give more fluids while increasing the rate of medication infusions. It didn't take long to reach the maximum dose of Levophed. With no response to the first drug, a second drip of Dopamine was started. Thankfully, after a few hours in the emergency room, Peter's systolic blood pressure stabilized above our goal of ninety.

Stabilized but still critical, it was time to admit Peter to the ICU. It's not unusual for septic patients to need blood pressure support. So it's not unusual for them to come to the ICU. But what was unusual was that Peter weighed over seven-hundred pounds.

There are not many people who weigh over seven-hundred pounds; admitting one in the ICU was rare. As soon as Peter entered our unit, we realized his unique situation was going to present a challenge. Our standard beds are designed to accommodate patients who weight up to four-hundred pounds. We had a problem, how were we going to properly care for this patient.

Our first call was to a company that provided specialty beds for special needs. We ordered a bariatric bed, a bed that is extra wide and built to accommodate extra large patients. Within a few hours the delivery was made. The company representative who delivered the bed would also assemble it. When he arrived, he surveyed the unit, and the area that the bed would eventually land. Our ICU does not have individual private rooms. Most of the beds are located in one large room and simply separated by privacy curtains. The layout, without walls, proved to be an advantage for the bariatric bed setup. The representative was glad to see that he would not have to deal with intrusive walls when preparing the area for the bed. He carefully inventoried the pieces of the bed, planned the assembly and proceeded with his work. He initiated his assembly in the hallway just outside of the ICU, and then astutely realized that this bed, once completely assembled, would not easily traverse through the various twists and turns between the assembly area and the location the bed would need to be for Peter to rest. After considering all options, he changed his building plans and decided to bring the bed into the unit in pieces and complete the assembly within the walls of the ICU. After completion of his job, he rolled this bed to the cubicle we call ICU 14 and assisted the staff as they transferred Peter onto his special size bed.

Transferring Peter onto his new bed created another challenge. Normally when a patient is transferred to the ICU, several nurses gather around. We use a slider board to assist with the transfer from gurney to bed. The slider board is a thin, but firm, piece of plastic with handles carved out of each side. The slippery aspect of the board allows the patient to slide easily over the sheets. The handles provide a place for the nurses to grasp and pull the patient from the gurney to the bed. With Peter, this was not going to be an option. The twenty-inch wide slider board would be lost under his extraordinarily wide torso. The routine plan with four nurses, two on each side, was not going to provide enough muscle strength to pull Peter from the gurney to the bed. Additional resources were needed to perform the simple task of transferring this patient to the bed. Four more staff members were called. Four orderlies responded to our call for help. Transferring Peter onto his bariatric bed required a total of eight strong staff members, four pulling and the other four pushing.

Once Peter was positioned comfortably, we continued to fight the detrimental effects that the infection was having on his body. We continued to infuse fluids through the multiple IV lines and titrated the drips to maintain our desired level of blood pressure. In addition to the most urgent need of blood pressure support, he also had wound care needs. Because of Peter's size, he was unable to perform comprehensive personal hygiene. In addition to the painful hip lesion, he had developed multiple skin ulcers on other various parts of his body. We found open sores in areas he had been unable to reach. These wounds required attention to prevent further infectious complications. The skin ulcers were weeping wounds that required dressing changes four times each day. Each time we needed to turn Peter to change these dressings, we again needed to activate the team of strong orderlies to assist. Four times a day, eight staff members gathered around his bed to turn, clean, change dressings, and change the sheets from under his oversized body.

We worked hard to support his infection-ridden body. We supported his blood pressure, we gave him antibiotics, we turned him side to side for wound care, and we talked and explained everything we were doing to him. We talked, but he didn't talk back. The sepsis had caused Peter to go into a barely-responsive stuporous state. Even though there seemed to be no obvious reason for him not to be able to talk to us, he wouldn't accommodate us with a return conversation.

Day after day, he lay in his special bariatric bed, motionless with his eyes closed as if he was oblivious to the world. Day after day, the team of staff came four times each day to perform this massive position change that was required for the wound care. Because he was not responding to our conversations, and because he was not talking back, many staff members, who came to the bedside to assist with the turning, erroneously assumed that he could not hear what they would whisper. A variety of comments would come from the bedside during the backbreaking events. Comments like "Look at that leg, it's as big as Jenny's entire body." "Looks just like the Pillsbury dough boy." "How can you tell where one roll ends and the next begins?" Many, too many, insulting comments were whispered while the team turned him back and forth. The unexpected sight of a huge belly, the puffy feet, and the stubby toes also elicited giggles and concealed laughter. All this while, Peter lay apathetically in the bed, at the mercy of the staff who were quietly making fun of the way he looked.

For weeks, we cared for Peter. Little by little, his blood pressure stabilized; little by little, the signs of infection cleared. But despite what looked like progress, Peter remained in that stupor for longer than we expected. We did lab work, x-rays, and scans, but nothing showed any physical reason why he couldn't respond to us. Tests showed that he had an enlarged heart. Heart failure caused by the excessive demands of his heart to keep up with the needs of his over seven-hundred-pound body. His lungs also showed some deterioration from years of obesity. His heart was weak and his lungs were struggling, but no tests showed a neurological reason for his obstinate mental state. So we waited … physical therapy continued to work day after day to strengthen his weakened muscles. The nurses worked hour-by-hour encouraging him to wake up and talk, but still no signs that Peter wanted to respond to our tender care.

Eventually, after his fever was normal, his blood pressure was back to baseline, and his wounds were healing, he started opening his eyes. At first, he would barely lift his lids and simply stared into the space surrounding his special bed. As we relentlessly talked and comforted him, he started looking at us, face-to-face. And then, with daily encouragement, he started nodding to questions, and off and on, he would mutter an occasional single word here and there. Finally, little by little Peter started opening up, but still in limited amounts. He would speak when spoken to, answer questions in short sentences, but never initiated any spontaneous conversations.

Six weeks after arriving in our unit, Peter's mentation returned to normal. He was finally communicating with each nurse who would care for him. We were happy to see him talking and visiting with his family members. Now he was ready to begin his journey home. But in order to get him strong enough to go home, we needed to get him out of the bed, work to strengthen his muscles, and reverse the damage that this life-threatening infection had taken on his oversized body.

We invited the specialty bed representative back to provide us with additional equipment that would help Peter return to his normal daily activities. One of the pieces of equipment the representative provided us with was a lift; a crane that could be used to get him in and out of bed. The apparatus looked just like the large hoist that is used in machine shops to lift engines out of cars. The nurses would position a pad under Peter's hips and back, fasten the four corners to the chains, and elevate him off the mattress. With a simple push of the seven-hundred pound basket, he would slide off the side of the bed, lower himself with the remote control, and land on the over-sized chair that had also been provided by the Bariatric Company.

We worked with him daily and eventually he was ready to be transferred out of the ICU. But unlike most patients, Peter remained in the ICU even after he was independent of the vasoactive medications and even after he had regained strength to assist with his own personal care. He remained in ICU because of his size. The equipment that was needed to care for him was so large that it would not fit in one of our standard rooms upstairs on the medical floor. Now he was awake, alert, and strong; he saw nurses come and go, while he sat in that same bed, day after day. While in the ICU, he built relationships with many of the nurses. He was becoming more talkative and friendly with all the staff. We don't usually have patients in the ICU who can talk and visit with the nurses. Unlike Peter, most other patients don't stay in the ICU long enough to become our friend. Peter became a friend; we got to know him as a person, not just a morbidly obese patient. He would joke with the nurses, and they would joke with him. He would wink at the nurses as they walked by the bed, and they would respond with useless threats of sexism.

We had fun with Peter, but we never lost site of our goal, to get him home. We worked daily to get him strong enough to go home once again. He looked forward to getting out of bed. He enjoyed taking control of the lift; we would help him in the sling and give him the controls. Peter would raise himself up until we gave him the all-clear sign. We would give him a push that he said was just like an amusement park thrill, and then he would lower himself into his special chair. Sometimes he would play with us, by going up and down a few times before setting down securely in his chair. That year, Peter spent Christmas in our unit. On Christmas Day, the nurses all brought food from home for our own Christmas dinner potluck. That year we shared our holiday meal with Peter. He enjoyed the pumpkin pie that I had made from my mom's favorite recipe. I remember him complimenting me, saying it was the best pumpkin pie he had ever eaten.

When it was time for Peter to go home, we didn't call the same ambulance company who brought him. We called another company who had an extra large gurney that could hold his over sized body. As Peter was rolled down the hall and out of the ICU, all of the nurses lined up to say good-bye. He gave hugs to everyone. Peter wanted hugs from all of his newfound friends.

During his four month stay in ICU, Peter lost almost one-hundred pounds. We provided him with education on healthy eating, a healthy diabetic life style, and some exercises he could do to continue the weight loss and strengthening his muscles. We tried to teach him some lessons that would help him in the future, help him stay healthy and stay out of our ICU.

During his stay in ICU Peter taught us some lessons as well. After he established confidence in the staff and developed a comfortable rapport with the nurses, he started sharing some concerns with us. He repeated many of the insulting comments that were whispered over his bed when the staff thought he was not lucid. He remembered the comments that were mumbled quietly by those who call themselves professionals. He shared with us his feelings of embarrassment during those humiliating dressing changes. He shared his feeling of disrespect from the staff that continued to laugh when they thought he wasn't listening. He relayed the insults he felt when the staff would comment on the need for the hoist because there were not enough muscles to lift him. And he taught us what it was like to be treated like a piece of meat instead of like a human being. He taught us some lessons, some lessons in discrimination, caring, professionalism and respect. He taught us that those large people we see out on the street are human beings and not lazy slobs who do not care about themselves. Once we got to know Peter, we all learned that obese people are real people. We all learned that these people have thoughts, a sense of humor, and feelings like the rest of us. Peter helped us to become professionals who care. Professionals who are careful with every word we whisper, and every action we perform. Peter helped us in our newfound ability to care for morbidly obese people with dignity and respect.

* * *

The next winter Peter was once again back in the emergency room. And, once again, he was admitted to the ICU. This time we knew exactly what equipment to order from the Bariatric Company. We had the bed delivered before he even got out of the emergency room. His special bed and all the needed care equipment was waiting when he arrived in our ICU. This time we knew exactly what equipment we needed to care for him and any other over-sized patient. We knew just what we needed to do and say in order to provide him with the same respect and professionalism that every person deserves.

Unfortunately, even though we knew how to provide support for Peter's oversized body, we were unable to provide the support to his failing heart. The second time Peter came to visit his friends in the ICU, we had to say a final goodbye. His failing heart could no longer keep up with the demands of his now almost eight-hundred-pound body. After just a few days of struggling to maintain life, Peter left us. But, most importantly, Peter left us with lasting memories and reminders of how to provide respectful care to all patients admitted to the ICU.

* * *

As the incidence of obesity rises in the United States, we see a corresponding rise in the number of obese patients we care for day after day. One more patient reinforced what Peter taught us. Lucy wasn't six, seven, or eight-hundred-pounds; she was a small three-hundred-and-fifty pounds. Three-hundred-and-fifty is easy for our

ICU beds to accommodate, so we didn't need to worry about ordering a special bariatric bed, but we did order a special wide bed that would allow for more freedom of movement. Because of her short stature, her weight had already caused a significant limitation in her movements. Because of the large, pendulous abdominal rolls, Lucy was unable to see a small sore that had developed under one of her abdominal folds.

Lucy came to our ICU from surgery after an I & D (incision and drainage) was performed. Usually, when an I & D is done, the surgeon makes an incision and drains the abscess by cleaning out the infectious drainage that was confined within the pocket of the abscess. After cleaning the pocket of infectious pus, the incision is closed and antibiotic therapy completes the treatment.

Unfortunately for Lucy, the surgical procedure was not that simple. When the surgeon opened the abscessed area, he found more than just a pocket of puss. He found necrotizing fasciitis. Necrotizing fasciitis occurs when bacteria attacks the soft tissue of the body. A wound occurs, bacteria invade the wound, and the bacteria eats away at the surrounding tissues. Lucy had a significant amount of bacteria-damaged tissue in the area of her abdomen and groin. The surgeon needed to remove a massive amount of tissue in order to prevent the bacteria from spreading to the rest of her body. Because of the excessive tissue removal during surgery, the incision could not be closed. The wound was so large, and the amount of skin and tissue removed was so significant, that the edges of the skin could not be pulled together. The surgeon had no choice but to leave the large gaping wound open.

I met Lucy the following morning in the ICU; she was about to have her dressing changed for the first time. Despite the major surgery that she had endured the evening before, Lucy was in a very cheerful mood. She was a big ball of happiness. She had big bright eyes and a smile that extended across her entire face. I could tell immediately that this lady had a great sense of humor. She greeted everyone as if they were entering her living room at home, not her

ICU cubicle. Yes, ICU *cubicle*—not an ICU *room*. Lucy did not have a room. She was in our ICU, the one that has most of the beds separated only by privacy curtains and not walls. But she was happy. She didn't care where she was; she was smiling and greeting all of her newfound friends with smiles and fun stories.

On this morning, we were expecting the surgeon, the infectious disease consultant, and the wound care nurse to meet at the bedside. They were to inspect the wound and make a plan of action. We, the nurses, were to have the dressing removed and the patient ready for their inspection. Two of us went to the bedside—the nurse assigned to Lucy and myself. I was the charge nurse that day. The nurse assigned to Lucy would remove the dressing and I would simply watch. I wanted to see the wound so I could communicate with the wound care nurse.

The removal of the dressing was more complex than we anticipated. We quickly discovered that I would not just be watching. The removal required one nurse to hold up the pendulous abdomen that obscured the wound while another nurse peeled back the tape and gauze. Once the two of us started our task, we discovered that the wound extended down and around the inner aspect of the thigh. Now we needed a third nurse to lift the leg, a leg that probably weighed at least fifty pounds. We needed one nurse to hold the belly, one nurse to lift the leg, and the third to dive into the wound with sterile gloves. Three of us were at the bedside, performing a procedure in an intimate area of a stranger's body. After what we learned with Peter, we were careful not to make any comments about the size of the body parts, or the difficulty in positioning, or the strength it took to lift a portion of her body. We were cautious about what we said to this lovely, lighthearted, fun-loving lady.

As the three of us worked in her groin, Lucy continued to smile in between her frequent whispers of "ouch." The dressing change proved to be a very painful experience. We made sure that she had as much pain medicine as we could give her; at least this would relieve some of the discomfort. We made sure that we explained every step to her in order to reduce her anxiety about what would happen next. And we made sure to talk to her throughout the entire procedure, so she could let us know when we needed to stop and give her a break.

We peeled the dressing off, the doctors examined the wound, the wound nurse consulted, and we developed a plan. Finally, we could reapply the dressing. Sounds easy, but it was not. Lucy's wound was the most enormous wound I had seen in all my years of nursing. It measured 60 cm long (almost two feet) from her left hip, across the outer edge of her large abdomen, and around the inner thigh. It was 34 cm (over one foot) wide and 7 cm. (three inches) deep on her thigh and 14 cm. (five to six inches) deep at the lower end of her abdomen. This large wound was going to require extensive time and effort to perform the dressing changes several times a day.

Our first goal was to address the pain. Because the wound was so deep, the internal tissues and muscles were exposed and therefore subject to any stimulation that we inflicted during the dressing changes. We provided Lucy with a patient-controlled analgesia (PCA) pump. This allowed her to push a button whenever she needed pain medication. We installed a large syringe of Morphine and programmed the pump so Lucy could administer pain medications whenever needed. Lucy was a large lady, so we set the PCA dials to allow for a large dose of medication. But that proved to be insufficient.

During the first dressing change, as we were gently packing her gaping wound, Lucy could not help but scream. "Ouch, I'm sorry." "OUUU" "Stop, Stop, Stop." "I'm sorry." More crying and screaming. The lighthearted Lucy was *apologizing* for her outbursts, but was unable to contain them. All we could say was "push your button, Lucy" and apologize as we continued, slowly and gently. As we performed this initial dressing change (that took three nurses over an hour to complete), the entire ICU had to endure Lucy's howls of pain. The privacy curtains did not protect the other patients and visitors from her suffering shrieks. We worked as gently and compassionately as possible and finally completed the task that we all found uncomfortable and painful.

As the charge nurse, I was delegated the authority to do what was needed for the unit and all the patients. I quickly realized that the ICU, with the privacy curtains, was not the place for Lucy. If she was going to have to endure painful dressing changes three times each day, the other patients and visitors should not have to endure them along with her. Our unit is set up with a few private rooms separated from the larger ICU. These rooms are usually used for isolation patients, but today I was going to make an exception. A private room would allow the nurses to close the door during the dressing changes and provide Lucy some privacy. The private rooms also have a large window that looks outside and a television that is not available in the cubicles. I was anticipating an extended stay for Lucy and felt that this young vital lady could benefit from these amenities that would allow her some sense of time. But moving Lucy down the hall was not going to be as easy as simply pushing her bed to a waiting empty room.

Lucy had been placed on an extra-wide bed. I suddenly realized that this bed might not fit through the door to the room of choice. What if it wouldn't? Do we leave her in the middle of ICU? Do we disassemble the bed and reassemble it inside the room? What will we do now? We measured the width of the bed and then measured the width of the ICU door. Luckily, the bed measured three quarters of an inch less than the doorway. Later that day, we moved Lucy down the hall into her new private room. That was where Lucy would reside for the next two months.

For the first few days, we did dressing changes three times a day. The new room, with a door that could be closed, allowed Lucy to cry out when she needed to. After the third day, we changed routines and started a state of the art wound device. The VAC, vacuum assisted closure device, uses foam pads to pack the wound. Then a plastic-wrap type dressing seals the wound, followed by suction tubing attached to a vacuum device. The concept is to allow the vacuum device to provide continuous suction on the wound; the constant suction promotes healing. The VAC would be maintained until the wound healed significantly and a skin graft could be done. The advantage of the VAC dressing over routine dressings is that the VAC dressings only needed to be changed three times each week, rather than three times a day.

For Lucy, this three-times-a-week procedure became a dreaded event, but less dreaded than three times each day. The dressing changes continued to be painful, but by bathing the wound with topical anesthetic before removing the old dressings and administering stronger pain medications, the dressing changes were tolerable. Not enjoyable, but tolerable. Every other day (the days of the dressing changes) she would become quiet and depressed, while on the opposite days she was happy and cheerful. Her moods were consistent with what she knew was planned for that day. Even though she tried to be her normal cheerful self, we could tell she had to try harder on the days the dressings were changed.

Lucy remained in the ICU for the entire time her wound was open. The dressing changes continued three times a week. The dressing changes alone required the undivided attention of three nurses for over an hour. This was a higher level of nursing care that could not be done on the medical floor when nurses have a team of patients. Because the wound extended from the abdomen, down and around the inner aspect of the thigh, one nurse had the job of holding the leg up while the others held the abdominal fold and dressed the wound. The nurse who was holding up the leg had to position herself on the bed and use her own arm as a prop for the large leg. The position of the elbow on the mattress and the leg perched on the nurses' hand allowed for that nurse to keep the leg off the bed for an extended amount of time. If the nurse would try to simply lift the leg, she would be tired and sore within minutes. This position, while rather invasive to a very personal area of the woman's body, allowed for a more tolerable means to the end. One day, I was the nurse leaning into the bed, positioned to hold Lucy's leg off the mattress; once again Lucy's sense of humor came to life. The conversation, of the three nurses and Lucy, developed into something similar to the *Vagina Monologues*. The *Vagina Monologues* are a stage comedy discussing what a vagina would say if it could talk. I hear the monologues are very funny. On that day, we had our own comedy, the *Vagina Monologues* in the ICU. After the dressing change, Lucy had us all laughing once again.

Most of our time with Lucy was cheerful, and most of the nurses maintained a professional attitude when it came to her size. Throughout the entire stay, I heard inappropriate comments only once. One nurse, who was doing the dressing change, while another was holding the leg, made a comment that I'm not sure Lucy even noticed. As she was leaning under the leg to secure the dressing to the inner thigh she said "Don't drop that leg, you'll knock me out."

Oh no, here we go again. Hadn't Peter taught us all to keep our insulting comments to ourselves? Hadn't that nurse learned from Peter that small comments could be painful? I immediately worried about what was going through Lucy's mind. "I know I'm fat, you don't have to remind me."

I quickly looked at her face to see if I could identify any expression that would give me a sign that she had heard that insulting comment. There was no expression on Lucy's face that told me she heard. Maybe I was the only one who that comment registered with. Maybe because I was more sensitive now, it hurt me more than it hurt Lucy. I hope so.

We continued her routine dressing changes, even got her out of bed walking around the unit with her vacuum device. Lucy enjoyed walking around and talking with all the staff. She was always upbeat and happy, and always found something nice to say.

One day when I was peeking in on her, Lucy seemed to be able to read my mood.

"What's wrong with your face?" she asked with a puzzled look on her face.

"Nothing's wrong with my face," I started, "why, what do you see?" I continued.

"It's not what I see, it's what I don't see." A short pause, as our eyes met she finished, "there's no smile." And we both laughed together.

During the time she was in our unit, all the nurses would often say that if they were having a bad day, they could go into Lucy's room and she would always have a smile for them. She would force them to smile back and that was just enough to give them the strength to finish a difficult shift.

After ten weeks of VAC therapy, the wound had healed enough for the plastic surgeon to plan the skin flap. As we were discussing this next surgery with Lucy and her family, someone asked where the doctor would get the skin for the graft. Lucy quickly answered for the doctor that she definitely had plenty of skin to spare. "Maybe he can take lots of skin and a little fat too," she joked.

Lucy went off to surgery and returned with a large dressing on the abdomen and a superficial dressing on the thigh where the doctor had removed the skin for the graft. After a short time recovering in the ICU, it became apparent that Lucy no longer needed the extensive nursing care that she once had. Now that the graft was successful, and the pain was controlled, Lucy was transferred out of our unit. But she wasn't done with us. Because we had all become friends with Lucy, many of us would stop by her room on the surgical floor just to say "Hello." When we would see her family in the cafeteria, they would eat with us. And on the day that Lucy was going home, her brother loaded her in a wheelchair and brought her back to the ICU so she could say good-by to all of her new friends before leaving.

* * *

Both of these over sized patients proved that they have oversized hearts and an abundance of friendship to give. Peter taught us a lot, not only about large size people, but what not to say when we think the patient isn't listening. Our comments, even though we think they are quiet and harmless, may cause significant grief for another. Obese people are not what many of us have in our stereotypical minds. But they are no different from the rest of us except there is more of them to love. Lucy did more than reinforce the lesson Peter taught us, she taught her own, even though you may have horrendous pain to endure, that shouldn't stop you from smiling and helping others to smile too.

Why is it that morbidly obese people are so friendly? Are they really overly friendly, or is it that many of us just never take the time to get to know them? Are they overly friendly because they have to work harder to have friends because of all of the misconceptions and stereotypes? Next time you see a Peter or a Lucy, think about your misconceptions, then think about the real person that is deep down inside. And, remember to think about what you say, mumble, whisper, or *think*.

CHAPTER 8

Give Me A Drink

Alcoholics often go through withdrawals while in the ICU,
requiring special care and attention.

Alcoholism is an illness, resulting from the daily consumption of alcoholic beverages. This regular consumption, day after day, results in a dependency. As the alcoholic becomes dependent on the drink, the drink causes not only psychological obstacles but also physical ailments. Psychological impacts include a craving to drink and this compulsion to drink often results in the alcoholic's inability to maintain normal daily activities. Jobs and families are often destroyed by the alcoholic's need for a drink.

The physical impact of the disease of alcoholism often results from the damage that occurs to the liver. This liver impairment results in a build up of body fluids and pressure in the circulatory system. Because of the close proximity of the esophagus to the liver, the blood vessels in the esophagus may become over distended and bulging. As the bulging blood vessels expand, they rupture causing bleeding. The bleeding causes either vomiting or loss of blood in the stool. This bleeding often becomes so severe that the alcoholic becomes weak from loss of blood and reports to the hospital for treatment.

Alcoholics are often admitted to the ICU when the bleeding is significant and the blood count is extremely low. The unstable condition requires close monitoring and immediate interventions. The first three days of the alcoholic's stay in ICU are spent focusing on replenishing the blood and identifying the source of the bleeding. Additional problems occur, usually on about the third day, when the body realizes there is no longer consistent alcohol intake. Once the alcoholic stops the daily ingestion, the body goes through alcohol withdrawals.

Alcohol withdrawals can result in delirium tremens, also called DT's. The initial signs of DT's are usually confusion. The patient will start forgetting where he is, maybe forgetting who the people around him are, and suddenly start repeatedly asking to go home. Despite the reassurance by the nursing staff that the patient needs to be in the hospital, the patient will start asking over and over to go home, not remembering why he is in the hospital, or even where he is. After the initial confusion, hallucinations occur. The alcoholic will start seeing and talking to things that are not actually there. Initially, the air vent on the wall may look like a bird up in the corner, and the garbage can may look like a basketball or a dog that needs to go outside. Then the hallucinations will progress to crawly things and people talking. The confusion and the hallucinations can cause significant agitation when the patient doesn't feel like the nurses are addressing his needs.

At the same time, the patient is experiencing these mental challenges; the physical effects will become more obvious as well. Early signs include shaky hands, and an unsteady walk. At first the shaky hands may not be noticed, but the patient will start to feel a little anxious. Eventually the nurse will notice that the patient shakes when reaching for a drink of water, or when feeding himself a meal. In addition, the patient will lose his balance when standing, and if not watched closely will stumble and fall. Confusion, hallucinations, agitation, and tremors present a challenge when it comes to caring for the alcoholic patient. This patient will be confused, will be trying to get out of bed, and will be pulling out any medical tubes that have been attached. He may be stumbling down the hallway, sometimes naked because he has removed all his clothes.

Our goal, the healthcare team, is to prevent the alcoholic patient from going through DT's, if possible. DT's, if severe, can result in seizures and death. To prevent the DT's, we administer benzodiazepines like Librium or Ativan. Benzodiazpines bind with the same receptors in the brain that had previously been binding with the alcohol. When the alcohol is eliminated, the brain receptors no longer have anything to grab onto, and the brain becomes irritable, thus causing the delirium, confusion and ultimately seizures that may cause death. The goal is to provide low doses of these medications to satisfy the brain and prevent the withdrawals while the patient receives the medical treatment for his physical problem.

If the patient does not admit to regular alcohol intake on admission, the healthcare providers will be alert to the signs within a few days. The signs of DT's usually start about the third day in the hospital. The delirium and the tremors signal the nurse to ask additional questions of the patient and the family to identify if this patient consumes alcohol on a daily basis. Usually the nurse will hear things like, "I drink a few beers every night after work." We usually double the amount that is offered as daily consumption. Three beers each night usually means a six-pack. If the patient admits to a pint of Vodka a day, we can assume that he drinks a quart. Alcoholics will usually admit to only about one-third or one-half of what they actually drink. It is usually the wife, or the significant other that clears up the amount and reports the true quantity that the alcoholic really consumes.

If we haven't been able to initiate the Benzodiazepines prior to the start of the DT's, then the dosages to control the DT's will be significantly higher than they would have been to prevent them in the first place. The confusion and agitation that these patients experience sometimes requires extremely high doses of sedatives. The increased amount of sedatives requires that these patients be monitored in the ICU because of the risks that these large doses carry. Frequent monitoring, frequent sedation, and an increased need for observation warrants an ICU bed for these patients. It's often a challenge to provide care for the patient and maintain their safety as they suffer through the horrifying DT's.

The family members often experience distress when they have to watch a loved one suffer through this painful experience. Having to see your loved one confused and "out of his mind" is not easy. Not only does he not know what he is doing, he doesn't know who anyone else is either. The safest way to treat the DT's is to sedate the patient through them, wait for them to pass, then back off on the amount of sedation, and wait for the patient to return to normal. Even though it sounds simple, it's not.

* * *

Kevin was 45-years-old when he came to us from the emergency room. Even though Kevin complained of abdominal pain, unlike the majority of the alcoholics, he had no signs of gastrointestinal bleeding. Kevin had not been eating much lately because it was the end of the month. He was homeless and he had run out of his monthly payments—he had run dry. Literally, Kevin had run dry. He had not had a drink in a few days. In addition to his pain, he was also complaining that he was shaky. He told the emergency room staff "I think I'm going through DT's."

Kevin had evidently gone through DT's before and knew what the initial feelings were. What did Kevin think we could do for him? What did Kevin want us to do for him? Because he was homeless, did he come to the hospital for a warm bed and a free meal? Did he make up the complaints of abdominal pain, just to be admitted? Did he know that if he came to the emergency room and told the staff that he was going through the DT's, that they would admit him? No one really knows what Kevin's plan was, but he ended up in our ICU.

I guess the emergency room doctor knew what he was doing when he admitted Kevin to the ICU. He admitted him with the diagnosis of abdominal pain and impending DT's. He knew what was coming, and he knew that it was coming soon. Unlike the others, Kevin didn't wait until day three to start his adventure through withdrawals. Because he had already been without his daily dose of alcohol for a few days, Kevin was already in the initial phase of withdrawal. Despite the sedatives that we started giving him as soon as he was admitted, his withdrawal came fast and hard.

Within twenty-four hours of admission, Kevin was confused.

"Do you know where you are?" A common question we ask all our patients to identify if they are oriented to their surroundings.

"Hell yes, I'm in a barn." He thought he knew exactly where he was. And if you had ever seen our ICU, all the beds separated by privacy curtains rather than walls, you might not disagree with him.

"Do you know why you're here?" Another question to determine if he was with us at all.

"Hell no, nobody asked me to come here." His language was another example of his street nature.

I tried to reorient Kevin frequently. I reminded him that he was in the hospital and reminded him of the town that he was in. But despite my verbal interventions and the frequent sedatives, Kevin started getting agitated in addition to his disorientation. He quickly started repeating his request for us to allow him to leave. Saying, "I got to go home," "Come on, let me up so I can go home," or even, "Hey, let me out of here so I can go home." Each of his requests were answered with reassurance and more attempts to reorient him.

"Where is home?" I would ask.

"You know," he would say as he looked around the room, "over there," and he would point to the other side of the ICU.

"You can't go over there, you need to stay here, in this bed." I would calmly reassure him.

Just as I thought I had convinced him to stay, he started pushing things away from the bed. The bedside table, with his dinner on it, went shooting across the floor. Kevin was climbing over the side rail in an attempt to get out of the bed, bare butt and all, but not before he pulled out his intravenous catheter. Now he was bleeding all over himself. Blood was dripping from his forearm onto the bed sheets and the IV fluid was dripping all over the floor. Immediately several nurses converged to help diffuse the commotion. I was trying to explain to him that he needed to get back into bed.

"No, I'm going home!" His voice was getting louder now.

Our goal, those of us who had congregated, was to confine this situation without causing stress on the other patients who were just feet away.

"Kevin, sit down please." I pleaded in a calm voice.

"Go to hell," was his answer to my polite request, as he stumbled a few steps toward the end of the bed. His tremulous hand grasped for the foot of the bed as he searched for his clothes.

"Get some restraints." I exasperatedly said to the nurse at my elbow. Restraints are soft fabric ties used to constrict movement by securing patients to their beds. We use them to prevent the patients from harming themselves. Restraints come in a variety of styles, depending on the needs of the patient. A vest restraint is used to keep the patient from climbing out of bed. Wristband restraints are used to secure the patients' hands to prevent them from pulling at or removing tubes. Restraints can also be tied to the ankles to prevent patients from kicking the nurses.

Patients in DT's, first of all, do not agree that they need to be in the hospital, because second of all, they do not realize what they are doing. Once the DT's start, there is no reasoning with the patients. For their own safety, restraints are necessary. We always try alternatives to restraints—reorientation, reasoning, closer observation. But when all other interventions fail, the use of restraints may be necessary for the patients' safety.

As Kevin stumbled around the end of the bed, several nurses remained close. Unfortunately, on that day, none of our male nurses were in the unit. How is it that they all seemed to have the same day off? Often men, confused men, will respond to the male nurse better than they respond to the female. Often confused patients think the male nurse is the doctor, and they figure the doctor has more authority than the nurse, so they follow their commands more readily.

We continued to try to talk Kevin into sitting on the side of the bed. If we could get him to sit down, we could then get him back into his bed safely. If we let him stand up and stumble around, it was only a matter of time before he fell.

"Kevin, sit here," as I patted the bed, "and I'll try to find your clothes." Coercion might work. I'd tell him anything I needed to get him back in that bed.

"I know they're here," as he took a short minute to look around. "Where the hell are my clothes?" He was yelling now.

Just as the nurse who was helping me reached for him, to try to coax him back to the bed, he swung his arm around a hundred-eighty degree to break loose of the grasp. He almost socked her on the top of the head, but her quick movement prevented any injury.

Kevin decided that to get his clothes was his only priority right now and if the nurses weren't going to give them to him, he would leave anyway. So, with his bare butt hanging out from behind the pale blue gown, his bare feet, still filthy from street living, and a blood stained forearm—Kevin was leaving.

None of us were going to get between his strong arm and the door. We needed reinforcements. "Call Code Help." I barked to anyone who would listen.

Code Help was announced on the public administration system when there is an event that requires immediate reinforcements. Code Help means that all big, strong men in the area are to respond. Security guards, housekeepers, engineers, nurses, orderlies, and any large man who is in the area will respond. Hopefully with an invasion of a large group of men, the person who is causing the commotion calms down. If that doesn't happen, the abundance of men will assist in subduing the person who is out of control.

As Kevin staggered toward the door, three tall men came through it from the other side. Two of them were wearing security uniforms.

I had remained close behind Kevin, ready to catch him when he fell because I knew that it wouldn't be too many more steps until he was on the floor. As he approached the door, and met the three coming toward him, he faced them adamantly.

"Sir, how can I help you?" asked one of the security guards politely. He knew immediately, as he entered the unit, why we had called the Code Help.

"I'm going home." Kevin tried to explain to him.

"No sir, you can't do that." More calmness came from the six foot two security guard.

"Like hell, I can't," and Kevin lurched toward the door that had just been closed behind the three gentlemen. Just as he moved one more step, he lost his footing and like an orchestrated play, each of the security guards grabbed an arm. That maneuver prevented Kevin from hitting the floor. He was able to regain his balance, as much balance as he had, considering the amount of sedation he had received, and the unsteady gait he was experiencing due to the alcohol withdrawals. Each of the guards kept their hold on Kevin and walked him back to his bed. The size of the guards was enough to intimidate him into submission. With the additional visual restraints of the guards, we were able to place a vest restraint on Kevin, and secure it to the bed so he would not be able to get up without assistance. Kevin continued to shout obscenities at us as we held his arm down on the bed to restart his IV and administered an additional dose of sedative.

Kevin had quickly entered the worse part of withdrawals. Despite the frequent doses of sedative, he continued to pull at his restraints in an attempt to get out of bed. He would bite at any tubing or device he could reach. And he would kick anything that came close to his bed. Within an hour, Kevin was in a vest, and had his hands and feet restrained to the bed to prevent him from injuring himself and anyone who came near enough to care for him. Despite the physical restraints, Kevin continued to yell obscenities until the sedative calmed him.

During this acute phase of DT's I was giving Kevin sedative doses every five minutes—one milligram every five minutes. This allowed me to continue to administer the sedative in small frequent doses, while continuing to monitor for effect. As soon as he calmed, I backed off with the medications. Then after a few minutes, he would wake up, yelling and fighting once again. The frequent dosing of sedatives, that was required to control Kevin's unsafe behavior, was consuming all of my time. Finally, I phoned the doctor to get an order to start a continuous infusion of the sedative. This continuous infusion would provide an even flow of sedative, just enough to keep Kevin safe, and I could give additional doses as needed if he had additional outbursts. The goal was to keep Kevin sedated until his body had a chance to go through the withdrawals, and to keep him sedated just enough to prevent seizures, and to keep him and the others around him safe from his delirious behavior. Kevin remained on the sedation infusion for several days.

* * *

Often, because the nurse works so hard to gain control of the patients who are out of control with DT's, once control has been achieved, she is reluctant to back off on the sedation. Too often, when the nurse hears from the previous nurse, during report, that the patient was still restless and confused, she will maintain the same level of sedation, without modifying the dose throughout her entire shift. Or she may increase the rate of infusion if the patient shows any slight signs of restlessness, because she knows how hard it was to gain control in the first place. It's important for the nurses to reduce the dosage to re-evaluate the patient's behavior, without allowing the patient to slip back into the dangerous behavior. When the patient stops showing any signs of agitation, restlessness, or confusion, the nurse will back off slowly and eventually discontinue the sedation.

I think that, too often, alcoholics remain over sedated after the craziness of the DT's are over. There is no set time that it takes for a patient to go through DT's. The length may depend on the amount of alcohol consumed on a daily basis prior to DT's. The more alcohol consumed, the longer the DT's. The length also varies for each patient, depending on liver function and a variety of other physical effects. But too often, in my opinion, some nurses continue the sedation too long after the delirium has passed.

Why? Either because of lack of knowledge or lack of initiative. The nurse may not have the knowledge and experience to realize that each day the dose should be reduced, and the underlying condition of the patient must be re-evaluated. Only after reducing the medication, can the nurse assess the patients underlying behavior and then decide if the same dose of continuous sedation is necessary. Or the nurse may not want to take the initiative to be an active care provider for that patient who was such a challenge to get under control in the first place. Some nurses may choose to maintain the same dose of sedation based on their own needs, not the patient's. It is easier to let the patient remain sedated; just in case he is not done with his DT's, than it is to spend time backing off on the dose, then administering additional doses to regain control. Sometimes, what I see is the same dose of sedation infusion continued for several days despite the fact that the patient lays in bed doing nothing.

ICU is expected to provide a higher level of care, and the nurses should be expected to provide that care. To maintain a patient on sedation because of lack of assessment is unacceptable. The nurse should re-evaluate the alcoholic patient daily just as she re-evaluates any other critically ill patient. The alcoholic patient, once under control, should be maintained on the least amount of medication necessary to prevent tremors, seizures, and injuries. Once under control, the nurse should assess the need for continued medication each day, and reduce the medication gradually until the patient can be taken off all sedation and start getting back to normal. To keep the patient sedated, just in case they are not done with the DT's, is not acceptable.

* * *

Kevin had been on his sedation infusion for six days when I was, once again, assigned to care for him. As I listened to report in the morning, I asked the nurse, "Why is he still on the drip?" Drip is what we call continuous infusions.

"I don't know, I guess because he is still in DT's," she responded.

"Is he restless?" my questions continue.

"Not for me, he wasn't," she answered quickly.

"Did you reduce the dose?"

"No."

"Did he wake up for you?"

"No."

I wanted to ask her next if she even tried to wake him, or if she even cared, but I decided to listen to the rest of her report and make my own assessment.

After the nurse had gone home, I did my initial assessment of Kevin. He would not respond when I called his name. He would barely wake up when I shook his shoulder. I reviewed the notes from the previous nurse, only to find that Kevin had been calm and sedated. He had not been restless and did not show signs of confusion. I reviewed the chart and found the sedation order to titrate the drip, based on the patient's agitation level. That's what I needed to know! I would reduce the sedation and reevaluate the exact amount Kevin needed to maintain his composure. I reduced the infusion from eight milligrams to six milligrams per hour. When the physician arrived for his morning rounds, he agreed with my plan.

"Go ahead, discontinue the drip and give him PRN doses if you need to." PRN is the acronym for a Latin phrase that means, "as needed." The doctor reviewed the orders to assure that I had a dose of PRN sedation for when I reduced the drip rate.

Throughout the morning, I continued to lower the drip rate as I monitored Kevin's level of consciousness. His mentation increased as I reduced the dose, but still he continued to sleep and was unresponsive unless I bothered him. By lunchtime I had the infusion down to a very minimal dose. I sat him up in bed and tried to get him to eat. He still could barely chew. As I fed him, I had to remind him to chew and swallow each bite. The liquids through a straw were about the only thing I could safely administer.

I continued to monitor him and by dinnertime, I had discontinued the sedation infusion. The restraints that were snugly attached when I came on duty in the morning were also removed. There were no signs of hallucinations, tremors, or any signs of restless behavior. Kevin was a sedated zombie. At the end of my shift, I reported my events of the day and reported that Kevin had been a perfect gentleman all day. I encouraged the night nurse not to give him any sedation so we could wake him up and get him moving in the morning. Today I was unable to get him moving but tomorrow I had big plans for Kevin.

When I returned in the morning, I was pleasantly surprised to see that Kevin had slept through the night and had continued to be that same perfect gentleman that I had left twelve hours ago. I was relieved, now I could pursue the plans that would get Kevin back on the road to recovery. I was going to get physical therapy involved in his care and start getting some strength back into those legs that had laid dormant in bed for over a week.

As always, I did my morning assessment. Today Kevin was talking. His speech was slurred, but at least he was saying words now. He was still under the effects of the sedation, but at least today his eyes were open and he was starting to act like a real person. Breakfast comes early in our unit. So as soon as my initial assessment was done, it was breakfast time. I sat him up for breakfast and started feeding him. Today he was chewing and swallowing without my constant reminders. Today he actually seemed interested in eating. Good—now we were progressing. I gave him the spoon, put it in his hand, helped him scoop some food and watch him try to eat as if I were watching a movie in slow motion. It took several minutes just for Kevin to move the spoon through the air toward his mouth inch by inch. By the time the spoon reached his mouth, most of the food that was on it to begin with was in his lap. We repeated this, bite after bite and Kevin made more of a mess than the average two-year-old child. But we had done this to him. We had sedated him to get him through his DT's. Now we had to be patient while the sedation wore off.

By lunchtime, I had Kevin in a chair. His legs were not as weak as I had expected, most likely because of his young age. I put the vest restraint on him, acting as a seat belt, because he would stand up or lean over to pick things up of the floor without concern for safety. His balance was still not back to normal. I was concerned that he would forget to ask for help, in his drugged state, and try to stand up and fall when I wasn't looking. Like breakfast, I watched as Kevin tried, inch-by-inch, in slow motion to feed himself. Often he would put the food on the spoon, lift it up and stop in mid air, as if he was sleeping sitting up and frozen in space. It would have been easy for me to simply take the spoon away and feed him bite by bite and allow him to sit limply in the chair. But instead, I placed my hand over his and slowly move his spoon-holding hand closer toward his face until he opened his mouth and found the resting spot for the morsels of nourishment. The massive amounts of sedation were leaving his system little by little; now we needed to build up his strength to get through the next phase of the recovery.

Our next task was to brush his teeth. His morning breath seemed about six-days-old. I provided him with the toothbrush, spread the paste on it and placed it in his hand. He looked up at me with a spaced-out look. His eyes were asking me, "What do you expect me to do with this?"

"Brush your teeth," I commanded.

He, once again, made a terrible mess with his weakened movements, but I finished the tooth brushing for him. We bathed, washed and combed his long, straggly blond hair, and shaved a week of whiskers off his face. As he was sitting up in the chair, belly full from lunch and body clean and shaven, his doctor made rounds.

"Wow, who is this guy?" he joked. "Doesn't look like the same man that has been here all week."

"We're getting ready for a party," I joked back. "Doesn't he look good?" I nodded for some reinforcements.

As Kevin sat up in the chair, we saw a smile on his face for the first time. He was still under the effects of the sedation that we had inflicted on him for such an extended amount of time, but now he was on his way to recovery.

"Keep up the good work," were the doctor's remarks as he wondered off to see his other patients.

Once up and around, it is not uncommon for these patients, in their post DT state, to sit in the chair, unable to move because they are in a drugged daze. They are unable to maintain their balance and be safe. And they are unable to bring their spoon to their mouth in a way that many of us don't even think about. The spoon remains suspended in mid air, moving slowly inch by inch toward the anxiously awaiting mouth.

That evening when Kevin was out of bed for dinner, a neurologist was visiting a nearby patient. I pointed Kevin out to him, as he was attempting to feed himself, his eyes half open and his hand in mid air. It seemed to be going in slow motion toward his mouth. I asked the doctor, who specializes in neurology, "What's up with this? Why is it that these guys do this? The suspended, slow motion movements."

"It's Ativanosis," replied the doctor.

"What?" I questioned this new disease that I wasn't familiar with.

"Ativanosis," he repeated. This time with a big smile on his face.

Now I understood what he was telling me. Ativan—the drug that we frequently use for sedation, and osis—meaning a disease, disorder, or condition. It was a diagnosis that he had just made up off the top of his head. But it made sense, because these patients are given such high doses of sedatives that, once they are done with the withdrawals from alcohol, they must go through withdrawals from the benzodiazepams. It takes time for the tremendous doses of drugs to get out of their system. As they wait for the treatment agents to leave their body, they slowly regain normal function.

We do it to them; we put them in the "ativanosis" state. But once off the DT-preventing sedation, it is up to us to help our patients get back to normal. Encourage them to start caring for their own needs. Allow them to get on with the beginning of a new life. Encourage them to get some treatment and support, despite the fact that we know many will be back in our ICU to go through withdrawals again.

That day, as I worked to help Kevin regain his normal life back, we spent a significant amount of time talking. I realized that he was not some scumbag, dope addict that was homeless because he blew his money on drugs and alcohol. I found out that Kevin had graduated from the same high school that I had. He went to college, had gotten married, and had a great job and a son. Several years later he started drinking and lost his job. His wife left him, took his son and all his money and he was left poor and on the street. He had only been homeless for less than a year, but had hit bottom rather fast. Kevin was a normal guy, a normal guy who was down on his luck.

Over the period of the next week, I took care of Kevin each day that I worked. One day he was ravaging through his belongings, looking for his baseball cap. We found his shoes, his pants and his shirt, which had all been diligently listed on the belongings sheet when he was admitted. But we found no baseball cap. Since it had been so long since he had been admitted, and not even sure if he had the cap when he came in, the only thing to do was to check the lost and found, just in case. We called, but no luck.

"Don't worry about it Kevin, we'll think of something," I tried to reassure him.

"But my hair is so long and messy." He was finally showing signs of normal concern about himself.

"I'll get you a cap, but not today." I had a plan, but for now I simply changed the subject. Kevin was probably thinking that I was just putting him off because I was one of those nurses who didn't care. One of those nurses who didn't want to hear about what he needed, but only wanted to worry about what I thought he needed.

The next day when I came to work, I brought him a baseball cap. The previous evening, when I got home from work, I went to my young teenage son's bedroom. He had baseball caps for every occasion, from a variety of teams, a variety of sizes, and a collection of old, useless hats from as far back as when he was five-years-old. I requested a donation that I could give to one of my patients who was homeless and had lost his cap. My son generously provided me with a choice of hats. I chose one that had some type of anonymous symbol on the front and took it to Kevin the following day. Kevin was grateful for the gift. It allowed him one more way to return to normalcy, to feel like himself again.

During the week that Kevin spent in ICU, attempting to overcome the sedation effects of the withdrawals, we worked on regaining his independence. Physical therapy worked with him daily to strengthen his gait and help him return to normal. Social services got involved. They worked with him to find an alcohol rehab program that would meet his needs, and found a shelter for him to live in when he was discharged. When Kevin was eventually transferred upstairs to the medical floor, where he would continue his recuperation, he looked like a completely different man than the one that had entered our ICU a few weeks prior. He looked like a normal guy, who had been through some hard times and who was down on his luck and could use some human caring.

A few days after Kevin's discharge from ICU, his doctor approached me. He complimented my care of Kevin. "Most nurses just want to keep giving these guys injections," he complained. "Why don't all the nurses wake them up and take care of them like you?" he asked.

My response was simply, "I don't know, I wish they did."

He went on, in a complimentary way saying, "I want you to take care of all my alcoholic patients, from now on."

"Thank you, but no thanks," I pleaded. And he understood my pleas, because he knew that caring for alcoholics during their withdrawals is one of the most challenging times for the nurse.

* * *

Alcoholics are one of the hardest patients to take care of. They may not be the most physically unstable patients in the ICU, but they can certainly be one of the most challenging. During the time that they are going through active DT's, they are confused, combative, loud, obnoxious, hallucinating, out of control, crazy, dangerous and at constant risk for seizures. Many nurses have been physically injured by the uncontrolled behavior of a patient experiencing withdrawals. These patients are one of the most frustrating and challenging for the nurse.

The standard care for these patients would be to provide enough sedation that would prevent the withdrawals. But sometimes, the patient is not forthcoming with the important information that will allow the physician to provide the needed medication to prevent DT's. When this occurs, the dreaded craziness starts, and it is the challenge of the nurse to prevent the life-threatening seizures that may occur during the withdrawals.

Once the DT's start, sedation is the only hope for control. Medicate them, to control their behavior and prevent seizures, and hope that we can control them before they injure either themselves or any one else. Sedate these patients to keep them safe, but don't over sedate them. Over sedation may cause unnecessary complications such as pneumonia and even respiratory arrest. Each nurse must balance on that fence between safety with adequate medication, and danger with unwanted complications. After control has been achieved, she must start evaluating the patient on a daily basis, to assess when the sedation can be reduced. As soon as the patient can control their behavior and be safe, we must back off on the sedation.

We work hard in the ICU, and sometimes the alcoholic patient makes us work harder than any other. During their acute state of delirium we are all in danger, the patient and the nurse. But danger also occurs when we, the nurses, don't reassess the need for continued sedation once the DT's are under control. And danger happens when we don't maintain safety for these patients. And danger occurs when we don't encourage the patient to obtain the support needed for continued success after discharge. It is important for us to remember the dangers of alcohol, not only for the patient and the nurse, but also for the family members who have to live with this disease daily.

The alcoholic patient presents a challenge for the nurses in ICU, but the patient has more of a challenge on a daily basis, than any of us will know.

They Are All VIP's

One day I reported to work, received my assignment and proceeded to the bedside for report. As I listened to report, I was told that the person lying in the bed was a VIP. Everyone knows a VIP is a very important person—someone who is special in some way to another person or to the organization. In this case, this patient was a retired physician and had served as a leader in the community for many years. Dr. Samuels was now in my ICU.

Today it would be my job to provide the best care for this VIP. As I planned my care for the patient, I considered all of his needs just as I would for any other patient. But for this patient I also had to make extra consideration for his privacy needs. Since Dr. Samuels had worked at the same facility that he was now a patient, I would have to deal with all of his physician friends who wanted to come visit and get medical updates on his condition. However, I needed to remember that Dr. Samuels was entitled to the same confidentiality that any other patient was permitted. I would also have to be prepared to give periodic updates to the hospital administrators. When VIP's are in the hospital, administrative staff members want to stay informed of the patient's status. So, I planned my care for this patient the same way I planned my care for all my patients—with the added responsibility of confidentiality and administrative updates.

It wasn't long into my day, when I noticed the Nursing Director was in the ICU. She didn't come to the ICU often, and I quickly realized that my patient's bedside would be her next location. As she approached cautiously, she inquired about Dr. Samuels' condition.

I provided her with an update: how his night went, how he was doing now, and what I anticipated for the day. I knew I could and should provide her with the medical information that she would maintain in confidentiality.

As I continued providing my normal level of care to Dr. Samuels, my next visitor was one of the hospital administrators. I allowed him to enter the room and express his best wishes to my patient. He didn't stay long, just long enough to let the doctor know he was there. As he left, I was sitting just outside the room. This high level administrator placed his hand on my shoulder and said "Thank you for taking such good care of him, he's very special to us."

"He's very special to us." That was his way of reminding me that Dr. Samuels was a VIP and I should give him the best care possible. At the time, I simply nodded my head and replied, "You're welcome." But after he had left the unit, I realized that I had not responded as I wished I had. When the hospital administrator thanked me for taking good care of this VIP and reminded me that he was special, I wished I had responded with, "*All* of my patients are very special to *me.*"

Just because Dr. Samuels was a retired physician, just because he was a highly respected member of the community, it was expected that I would provide a different level of care for him. The truth is, that I provide the best care I can to all of my patients, no matter who they are. I "take good care" of all of them.

I provided the best care I could to Dr. Samuels over the next few days. But, the care I provided was no different from the care that I provide to all my patients. I gave one of my son's old baseball caps to the homeless patient who lost his. I gave a piece of pumpkin pie to the morbidly obese patient because it was Christmas. I attended the funeral of one of my young patients with whom I bonded, and I do this because it is my nature to provide the best care to all of my patients because they are all VIP's to me.

CHAPTER 9

Dignity or Dress

*All patients are stripped of their clothes. How do we maintain
dignity for those in that skimpy gown?*

When a patient rolls into ICU, several nurses converge onto the
site of arrival. If a stranger was watching, it might look as if buz-
zards were swarming in for the attack. The team, usually two or
three nurses, depending on who is not immediately occupied with
other tasks, will slide the patient off of the gurney and onto the
more comfortable bed. The first thing we do is strip them naked.
Any clothes that may have survived the emergency room visit will
now be history; off with the socks, off with the trousers, even off
with the underwear.

The primary nurse, who will be responsible for this patient, has
previously received a report over the phone to alert her to the condition of the patient. The phone report, from the nurse in the emergency room, or whatever floor is transferring this patient to us, would
include the medical history of the patient, the problem the patient
is experiencing currently, and the treatments the doctors have decided to initiate. Immediately when the patient rolls in on the gurney, the other nurses in the unit will converge at the site of arrival.
Teamwork is vital for survival in our high-level care area. No one
would expect that one nurse would be responsible to initiate critical

care treatment single-handedly. As the primary nurse prepares her plan of attack, reviews the physician's orders and assesses the patient, her helpers set out to make her job easier.

None of us like to get admissions. We all prefer to come to work, start our shift with two stable patients, the key word being stable, care for them all day or night, and give report to the same nurse who gave us report twelve hours ago. That is a nice day in the ICU. Unfortunately, our goal is to restore the health of our patients. Once we do that, they move out of our unit to the medical or surgical floor. Then there is always another more critical patient waiting to come. The nurse, who has just transferred her stable patient to the floor, now receives the first incoming unstable patient. That nurse becomes the primary nurse, while the others assist her in the settling of the patient.

We work in tandem, settling the patient. We attach a variety of wires to every patient in order to provide the observation that is required. Each of these wires allows us to monitor a specific parameter, EKG, oxygen level, blood pressure, pulse. In order to attach the wires, we first need to purge any obstructions, anything that will hinder our ability to monitor and assess. Shirts, pants, socks are all considered obstructions.

* * *

Byron, upon arrival to the ICU, was grumbling and frowning at the variety of female nurses grabbing at him at various parts of his body. One nurse was taking off the pants and socks. Another was shaving the thick curly hair from his chest in small round areas in order to attach the cardiac monitor. And the third was attaching the blood pressure cuff to the right arm followed by the oxygen saturation monitor to a finger on his left hand.

"But why do you need to take everything off?" Byron questioned as his pants were being tugged away.

"Byron," I started. He looked like a guy with a sense of humor. "When you were in the emergency room, did they ask you to sign a piece of paper called Conditions of Admission?"

He nodded affirmatively and I continued. "That paper said you agreed to be admitted to the hospital and receive treatment?"

"Yes," he answered, with a puzzled look on his face.

"Did you read the fine print?" I paused to give him time to ponder my next question.

"No," the puzzled look now became a look of fright.

"The fine print said that you give up the right to be modest, and you give permission for anyone and everyone to peek at any and all parts of your body."

With this, we all enjoyed a laugh and it lightened up a stressful situation for the man who was being admitted after having his first heart attack at the age of thirty-nine.

"Now, off with the underwear," I concluded as he grudgingly let loose of his last piece of clothing.

* * *

We explain to our patients the reason to remove all clothing. As soon as they enter the ICU and the barrage of nurses approach, we start talking. Each nurse explains the piece of equipment that she is attaching. The reason for removal of personal items will be clarified. "Because of all of the tubes and wires, we need to have access to your entire body." We have nice, thin, pale blue gowns that every patient is allowed to wear. They certainly are not fashionable, but are very functional.

With the entire back open, the gown is placed on the front of the patient, both arms are threaded through the sleeves and one tie is secured behind the neck. With the large opening in the back, this gown allows any and all medical personnel to lift the gown from the front and view any portion of the body required. Remember, these patients are in ICU and ICU nurses like to be in control; we want to be able to see any, and all parts of the patient at any and all times. But besides making our job easier, it would be uncomfortable for the patient to sleep in their clothes.

Honestly, it is important to allow our patients opportunity to maintain their dignity, but allowing them to keep their clothes on won't do it. We allow the patients to keep their dignity by providing them with some sense of privacy, after they are naked. We try hard to maintain privacy while in the ICU. Our unit is one big room, with areas designated for beds and separated by privacy curtains. This makes privacy and dignity more of a challenge than some units. In newer ICU's, each bed is in its own private room enclosed with real walls.

Many of our patients are in the ICU because they require a higher level of observation. This large open unit allows for all of the patients to be seen from various locations throughout the unit or from the one central nurses' station. It also, however, allows for all the patients to be seen by anyone who chooses to walk past the end of their bed—staff, visitors, and even other patients. The only way to maintain total privacy is to keep the curtains pulled totally around the bed at all times. If the curtains are pulled completely around each bed at all times, the nurse cannot see that patient. Thus the goal of increased observation is not possible.

Many of our patients are in ICU for increased observation because they are not cognizant. Many, either because of their disease process or because of the medications we administer to them, are not aware of their surroundings. Many of our patients are on life support, sedated and are not aware if the patient next to them is naked or not. But the family who comes to visit daily is certainly aware of the neighbor who may or may not be lying in the bed in a dignified manner.

ICU is a scary place, the place where the hospital puts those who are really sick and those who need to be watched closely. Visitors must sometimes walk past several patient cubicles to get to their own family member's bed. On the way, the visitor may see a little old lady pulling off her clothes, but they try not to stare.

They might see the man who is delirious and shouting obscenities. As he kicks his legs, his pale-blue gown becomes bunched up around his chest, exposing the entire lower half of his body. The visitor will politely turn away. Visitors may also turn their heads toward the bed of a dying patient. Although tubes and machines are obscuring the view of the patient, several grieving family members can be seen surrounding their loved one.

Maintaining dignity at each of these bedsides is a challenge, a never-ending laborious task. The nurse must maintain the dignity of each of these patients, the demented, the delirious, and the dying. She must consider those who will be visiting the unit as well. There are so many opportunities for each patient to lose their dignity, whether it is due to their mentation or sedation or situation, the nurse must never loose sight of the goal—even though we strip them naked, we need to maintain dignity. We need to care for these critically ill patients and keep them safe; sometimes we need to keep them safe from themselves.

* * *

Annabelle came to our ICU from an assisted living community. Her son brought her to the hospital because she was having difficulty breathing. Annabelle was admitted with a diagnosis of pulmonary edema. Pulmonary edema is an acute onset of fluid in the lungs. Unlike pneumonia that is an infection, pulmonary edema is simply an excess of fluid in the lungs. Diuretics, that rid the body of excess fluids, are often used to treat this ailment. Unfortunately for Annabelle, she also had high blood pressure that required a continuous infusion of an IV antihypertensive medication. Because of the frequent monitoring of her blood pressure during the infusion, she was admitted to the ICU. Her son informed us, at the time of admission, that at the age of eighty-six Annabelle suffered from dementia. Dementia is a disease that affects the elderly and results in loss of memory. Often short-term memory is affected more severely than long-term memory. Many patients who have dementia can tell factual stories about their younger years, but cannot recall what was said to them five minutes ago.

Several nurses settled Annabelle into the ICU, as usual. After being tucked into bed with monitoring devices securely attached, she seemed comfortable. Her blood pressure was being monitored every fifteen minutes as we titrated the level of medication needed to control her hypertension. Annabelle was in one of the beds located exactly in the center of our large ICU. It wasn't long before she realized that she wasn't in her normal area of recognition, and she was not in her own clothing. As soon as the nurse turned her back, Annabelle was stripping herself naked. With her right arm free and bare, she waved the pale blue gown that was hanging from her left arm over her head. Totally exposed, Annabelle's next task was to get out of that bed.

As I approached the bed, she looked up at me with helpless eyes. "Dear, can you help me?" she pleaded.

"What are you doing?" I inquired gently.

"I need help, I need to get out of here."

"Do you know where you are?" As I immediately started to re-dress her bare body, I needed to establish if she was oriented.

Again she looked around as if she was seeing the area for the first time. "No."

"You're in the hospital." I reassured her, as I realized she had no idea as to where she was.

A look of surprise came over her face. "Oh, thank you." She smiled as if I had just lifted the weight of the world off her shoulders.

I helped her put her gown back on. She thanked me again and laid her head down on the pillow. Five minutes later, as I was walking past the bed, Annabelle, once again, had her gown draped over only one shoulder and all of her sagging body parts were flashing for any available eyes to view. This time she was almost out of the bed, legs between the foot board and the side rail, and she was on her way to somewhere else, somewhere she had in her own mind. Once again, we went through the same conversation we had just finished a few moments ago. After I reminded her that she was in the hospital, she thanked me but this time the smile on her face was not as convincing. It seemed as if she was thinking that perhaps I really didn't know what I was talking about. That look of doubt was in her eyes and the expression on her face told me that she was pacifying me by getting back into bed, but in her own mind, she knew that I didn't have a clue as to where I was.

This time, I didn't leave her bedside. I simply turned my back and waited about thirty seconds. As I twirled one-hundred-and-eighty-degrees back toward her, she was once again pulling at the gown. Frustration consumed my thoughts, *how was I going to keep Annabelle covered and safely in bed?* As soon as I left her side, she was stripping and squirming. No amount of reminders, reassurance and redressing was going to work with Annabelle. I needed to consider her dignity while maintaining her safety. I'm sure she wasn't aware that others were going to peek at her naked body each time she stripped and climbed to the foot of the bed. Each time she pulled the gown off, she seemed to wrap it, dangerously, around another part of her body. My only option and my last resort was to use restraints. We try not to restrain patients, but when all alternatives have been exhausted, restraints are used to keep the patient safe. The vest restraint, like the gown, goes on backward with the opening in the back. The back has Velcro to secure the closure, and two tie straps that secure the patient to the bed, like a seat belt.

I asked one of the other nurses to keep a close eye on Annabelle as I went to the supply closet to get a vest of the appropriate size. As I returned to the bed, my co-worker was once again redressing Annabelle and securing her position in the bed.

"Annabelle, I have something here for you."

"Oh thank you dear." She smiled with appreciation. This time, I could only imagine that she was thinking that I had finally come to my senses. I was going to help her get out of this predicament that someone had left her in.

"This will keep you warm and safe," I explained.

She helped me thread each of her arms through the vest arm-holes. She sat up in the bed as I secured the Velcro across her back, and then watched as I tied each strap to the respective side of the bed frame. She watched attentively and once again thanked me for my help. With the help of the vest, I was able to secure Annabelle's clothes, maintain her dignity and provide for her safety all at once. Annabelle was not able to remove her gown, now that the vest overlaid it, and she was not able to climb to the foot of the bed with the safety straps secured. Annabelle was safe and covered, and I was able to leave her bedside knowing that I would not return to see a bare body on the floor. Annabelle continued to ask for help, from any and everyone who walked by her bed. This time she asked for help to get out of the bed. "Can you help me? I can't get out." Each nurse would respond with some variation of "You can't get up right now," to "You're in the hospital," to "You need to stay in bed." Each time, Annabelle would smile and thank the nurse for her help. Annabelle was content, and so was I that she was not naked on the floor.

* * *

Like Annabelle, many of our patients are restrained. Dignity and restraints don't often go hand in hand. Dignity, to maintain self-esteem, to feel good about ones self, is not easily done with the use of restraints. Restraints often reduce a patient's self-esteem. When a patient is tied down, in any manner, it eliminates their ability to provide any self-care and does not allow for any self-esteem or dignity.

Imagine being in an accident and losing consciousness, or going off to surgery and after either of these events, waking up in a strange place. You are now sedated, still sleepy and awaken with a large tube in your throat. You have been placed on a ventilator because you are not able to breathe unassisted. You hear noises, bells and alarms ringing in your ears. As you barely awaken, you choke and cough, something is caught in your throat and causing you to gag. Your first instinct is to remove the obstruction, the irritation that is in your throat. The nurse grabs your hand and tells you not to touch your face or the tubes. Within another minute, you doze back to sleep and once again a cough initiates your hands to move instinctively toward your intrusive tubes. The nurse cannot trust you to keep your hands away from your lifesaving tubes during these hours of uncertainty, so she secures them to the bed. She does this for your safety, but you are in and out of consciousness and not fully aware of the reasoning.

Now you are half-awake, unsure of where you are, unsure of why that large annoying tube is in your throat, and you can't move your arms. Your wrists have soft bands, like handcuffs, attached to the sides of the bed. You are sedated, your mind is unclear, and perhaps you don't even speak the same language as the nurse who is talking across your bed with her co-worker.

How would you feel? Would you have your dignity intact?

* * *

The nurse deals with complicated situations daily. The patients in the ICU have a variety of tubes and a variety of machines to support normal body functions. The nurse must be in control of each of these tubes and machines that assist with the bodily functions of each of her patients. When a patient is not one-hundred percent cognizant, their actions may hamper the attempts of the health care team to treat their medical problems.

The nurse works hard to assure no interruption of the treatment options occur, whether it is by taking away clothes in order to access the entire body or by restraining the patient to keep her clothed in bed, or securing the hands to keep the sedated patient from pulling out lifelines. The nurse must maintain control in order to make sure that the critically ill patients are treated and safe. The nurse meets challenges on a daily basis. Challenges of many kinds, some are stressful—dealing with death, and some are frustrating—dealing with dignity. But she must never compromise the dignity of the patient, whether it is clothing or restraints, just to maintain control.

CHAPTER 10

Where Do They Go?

*Where do we discharge the homeless when
they have no home to go to?*

When a patient comes into the emergency room, they receive treatment. It doesn't matter if they have insurance or money or not. There are laws that protect the poor. Any person has a right to medical care. If the emergency room personnel turn away a patient because of lack of ability to pay, that hospital may be fined. So, any person who comes to the hospital for care must be treated, regardless of ability to pay.

Wintertime is a difficult time for many, but is especially difficult for the homeless. Many homeless have to search daily for a warm place to sleep. I often wonder if the homeless go to the emergency room with some non-specific complaint, because it's easier than finding a warm place to sleep. Not being an emergency room nurse, I am not aware of all the visits that occur. I only hear some of the stories. On really cold nights, some homeless people seem to suddenly develop un-diagnosable aches and pains. Usually these nonspecific complaints are just enough to require attention until the sun comes up again and it's warmer outside. Sometimes they receive an x-ray, a warm meal, a bath, and then they are on their way. Off to the streets to find yet another place to keep warm for the following night.

Randy came to the emergency room, one winter evening, complaining of a sore foot. A sore foot was enough to get him a bed in the warm emergency room for that cold winter night. He gladly unveiled his sockless feet from his worn shoes to allow the nurse to assess the problem. It was hard for the nurse to see what he was pointing to when she peered over his dry blackened feet. The dirt was caked onto each of his feet, obstructing any view of any apparent problem. The nurse encouraged Randy to indulge in a warm foot soak. She explained that soaking his feet in a hot basin of water would help warm them and help her to see the sore area better. Randy was happy to be pampered for a short time with the soothing water. After a few minutes of soaking, the water quickly turned to mud. Randy didn't want to remove his feet until the water cooled, the warmth was comforting. A second basin with more fresh hot water was provided with no objections from Randy.

As he withdrew his feet from the second tub, the source of his complaint become obvious. His right foot was considerably larger than the other, and the entire side of the foot was fire red. It appeared that Randy had a significant infection brewing on the foot, that he had simply reported as being sore.

After examination by the emergency room physician, it was obvious that Randy had a nasty infection of his entire foot. He reported that he had stepped on some kind of sharp object a few weeks prior. He assured the doctor that he had tried to keep it clean, but considering his living situation, that was not an easy task. His entire foot was exhibiting the signs of a roaring infection. Because infections can spread throughout the body and cause considerable illness, it was decided that intra-venous antibiotics were the treatment of choice. Randy was going to be admitted to the hospital. He would get that warm bed that he came searching for. He would get that warm bed for more that just one night, he was staying for several nights.

Once the decision to admit Randy was made, another decision—what to do with his belongings—had to be made. When Randy limped into the emergency room, he left his shopping cart outside the entrance. That shopping cart contained all of his worldly possessions. Upon learning that he would be admitted, he needed to be assured that his belongings would be kept safe. There was no space in the hospital rooms for the entire contents of the cart and there was no designated area that could store his belongings for an indefinite amount of time. Randy insisted that he be able to take his cart to his room with him. He was standing firm, arguing that in the cart was everything he owned, and many of the items were key to his survival. He even suggested that rather than compromise the security of his belongings, he would refuse treatment and return to the street with his possessions. It was becoming obvious that Randy knew what he needed to survive and he had to stand firm in order to get what he felt he needed for survival. But Randy was not out on the streets now; he was within the confines of an organization that had rules and regulations, not the free and clear land of the homeless. After some strong negotiations, Randy agreed to call his older sister Bobbie, who lived locally, and asked her to come pick up his things. Bobbie came, picked them up, and offered to store them in her garage until Randy was discharged.

After securing his belongings, Randy was admitted to the medical floor for continued antibiotic therapy. Randy, who had a history of heavy smoking, soon became restless in his hospital room. The no-smoking policy was a rule Randy did not want to follow. There was no smoking allowed throughout the entire hospital, even the staff must go to a smoking shack that is fifty feet away from the building. Despite the use of a nicotine patch, after a few days of not smoking, Randy was becoming more and more anxious. He seemed to be happy to be in the hospital, but angry about not being able to indulge in one of his addictive habits.

One evening, Randy decided he was going to leave the hospital in order to have a cigarette. He informed his nurse that he would be going out to smoke and would return when he was finished. The nurse instructed him that smoking was against hospital policy and tried to encourage him to change his plan. But Randy insisted that he had rights, and it was his right to smoke—he was not breaking any laws and he was going out of the building to have a cigarette. As his nurse tried repeatedly to convince him to stay, the conversation escalated and the confrontation became loud. The charge nurse stepped in to try to resolve the highly volatile exchange. She too tried to reason with Randy, but his hardened personality was hindering any amicable negotiations. She reiterated the hospital policy about no smoking. But Randy didn't seem to care about any policies. Every time the rules or policies were explained, it seemed that Randy would get more and more adamant about his right to smoke. Once it seemed that the battle was being lost, the charge nurse informed Randy that he would be allowed to leave. But, she explained that he should sign a form stating that he was leaving the hospital against medical advice (AMA) and his intravenous line would need to be removed and he would be discharged.

When a patient decides to leave the hospital before the physician decides it is safe to be discharged, that patient must take responsibility for his own health. The patient must acknowledge that any medical issues that may arise as a result of lack of treatment are his responsibility. The patient must sign a form stating that he is leaving hospital against the advice of the medical staff.

With this information, Randy became even more agitated; he started yelling at the nurses, obscene language could be heard throughout the unit. The nursing supervisor was called for additional support for this out of hand situation. The supervisor was on her way to the scene when she heard Code Help announced over the public administration system.

In this case, Code Help resulted in about five men rushing to the scene, at the same time that the nursing supervisor arrived. Randy was immediately aware that he had gone beyond acceptable behavior. Randy was not willing to sign out AMA, so he reluctantly agreed to stay in the hospital for continued antibiotic therapy. The alternative would be to stop treatment and risk losing his entire foot due to the infection. He returned to his room and remained relatively quiet the rest of the night. With only a few complaints and a few obscene comments, the nurses were able to appease him.

The next day Randy, once again, decided that he urgently needed to leave the hospital to have a cigarette. He quickly escalated into another rage. This time he was not only yelling but he was also acting in a threatening manner toward the nurse who was desperately trying to negotiate with him. He was raising his arms, as if to strike her and following those aggressive moves with a raising of his middle finger. When the Code Help was called to de-escalate the manic behavior, Randy quickly agreed to calm down and abide by the hospital policies. This time, however, the supervisor decided that this patient was more time-consuming than the nurses on the medical floor could handle and he was transferred to the ICU.

Prior to arrival to the ICU, the floor nurse gave a report to the receiving ICU nurse. The report included all of Randy's physical problems, medications, lab values, treatment plan, and an explanation of what had happened over the past few days. The nurse had reported that Randy seems to be very manipulative and when he did not get his way, he would act out. Randy was not being transferred to ICU because his medical condition warranted a higher level of care, but he was being transferred because he was simply too big of a hassle for the floor nurses to deal with.

In the ICU, the nurses only have two patients. California law requires this, because of the higher level of care. Not only are patients transferred to the ICU because of their need for a high level of assessments, interventions, and monitoring due to their critical physical condition, but also sometimes they are admitted to the ICU simply for increased observation, or for care that takes more time than the floor nurses have to give. Time-consuming interventions like calming, de-escalating, and watching closely are not possible on the medical floor when the nurse has four, five or six other patients. The closed rooms on the medical floor also prevent close observation, unlike the open ward setting in the ICU that allows everyone to watch anyone.

Randy was a behavior problem on the medical floor. The nurses could not provide the time-consuming attention and the constant de-escalating that he demanded, so he was transported by gurney to our unit. As he entered the unit, he was scanning his new surroundings. He could see immediately that this would not be a quiet semi-private room with a window and a television like he had upstairs. But, he had lost those privileges and would be sentenced to a stay in the ICU until he could prove that he could behave. It seemed as if it was punishment for Randy, punishment that he brought on himself when he stepped over the line and acted inappropriately. He was admitted to one of the ICU beds in the middle of the wide-open unit. No window, no phone, no television to watch, only nurses, and monitors and machines to listen to.

Randy settled into his bed, looked around and said, half jokingly, "Can I smoke here?"

The nurse, because she knew of his previous behavior, took a supportive compassionate tone of voice. "Do you see the oxygen on the walls?" No answer was necessary as Randy's eyes scanned the area. "Not only is it against hospital policy, but if you light a cigarette in here, we'll all blow up." A short pause was followed by "There will be no smoking, correct?"

"O.K. you're the boss." Now he was a little patronizing, but for now, he was cooperating and remaining calm. And just to make sure there would be no smoking, the cigarette lighter that was in his belongings was removed from the area and placed in a safe place in the charge nurse's office.

It was explained to Randy that he had been transferred to the ICU so we could watch him a little closer. His behavior on the medical floor was inappropriate and he would now remain in the ICU for the higher level of observation. At first, Randy seemed to think that this was a good idea. He liked the activity in the unit. He seemed to like the constant busyness that walked past his bed every few minutes, and he was entertained. But after a while, he started getting bored. Newspapers, outdated magazines and the daily activities of the staff could only keep him entertained for a short time. He started getting restless. He no longer had control of his situation. Out on the street, control is imperative for survival, but in our unit, Randy had lost control—*we* were in control.

Randy had noticed that at each end of the unit, we have a private room. These private rooms are used for patients who require either isolation or a quiet environment for medical purposes. Each of these private rooms has a television and Randy decided that he wanted to be moved into one of those rooms. The nurse explained to him that the patients currently in those rooms needed to be there for a specific reason, but instead of a television, we could bring a VCR player, on a cart, to Randy's bedside and he could watch videos. That would help pass the time.

When Randy's doctor made rounds, we discussed his plan of care. We were informed that the doctor wanted to provide Randy with continued intravenous antibiotics. If Randy had a home, we could discharge him with some home health care and a nurse who could come to his home to provide the intravenous antibiotics twice a day. But, Randy's living situation presented a problem; he had no home, and he had no access to home health nursing. So, this challenge meant that he would be staying in our hospital for the duration of his therapy.

A few days later he watched one of the patients be transferred out of one of the desirable private rooms. When his doctor came to see him on that day, he convinced the doctor to move him into that room. The doctor obliged by writing an order in the physician order sheets "Please place patient in a private room." Randy had manipulated one more person into doing what he wanted.

When in nursing school, we learn that the nurses are to follow physician orders. We also learn that the nurse is not to carry out the physician order if it will harm the patient. If the doctor writes an order for the wrong dose, the nurse should not give that dose. If the doctor writes an unsafe order, the nurse should question the order before blindly abiding by the directions. This order did not have any unsafe component to it, but the nurses didn't really want to carry out that order. The nurses didn't want to allow this patient to have the private room, it seemed as if that would be a reward for his inappropriate behavior. But for now there were no other patients who needed the private room so Randy was moved and the television was used to pacify him.

After a few days, we admitted a patient who required the private room for isolation. We had no choice but to move Randy back out into the general population of the ICU. We brought the VCR to the bedside, assured that he had a variety of movies, and made every possible accommodation for his privacy that he felt he lost when moved out of the room.

It didn't take long for him to show that he was going to try to take control once again. Once again, he started asking, at first, and then demanding that he be allowed to leave the building to smoke. "I have rights, you know," was his support for his argument for smoking. We agreed that he had rights, but smoking was not allowed in the hospital and he would not be allowed to leave to smoke and come back in the hospital at his leisure.

As Randy became more agitated, he was pacing around his bed and threatening to sign out AMA. We phoned the social worker, Gary, to come assist us with his outburst. Perhaps Gary could talk to him and convince him that treating his dangerous infection was more important than having a cigarette. Gary spent some quality time with Randy. The two of them discussed his plan of care and the importance of the antibiotics to cure his infection. Randy tried once again to negotiate a compromise. He would stay, continue his antibiotic therapy and not sign out AMA if the nurses would allow him to go outside, to the sidewalk and let him have a cigarette two times each day. Gary agreed to discuss this option with the nurses if Randy would calm down and wait for a decision.

I was in charge in the ICU on that day. I was the charge nurse that the social worker came to discuss this compromise with. As soon as I listened to Gary's suggestion, I immediately thought, *how ludicrous, who would expect a nurse to leave her other critically ill patient while she sat on the sidewalk and watched that manipulative brat smoke a cigarette.* My response to Gary was "I don't think so, that is not an option."

"But consider it," he replied, "If we let him smoke, only twice a day, he will stay for his treatment." Gary was arguing Randy's side. He didn't have a clue as to what the nurse would have to do to accommodate this simple request.

"We don't have time to sit on the sidewalk while he smokes." I continued my argument. Then I turned the tables. "Why don't you commit to taking him outside for a cigarette twice a day." I suggested.

"I don't have time for that, I'm too busy with my caseload," he countered.

Was he suggesting that he was busier than the nurses? Was he insinuating that we were not busy? What made Gary think that we could leave our other patient, who may be unstable and need minute-to-minute attention, to accommodate this ridiculous request, but he could not? Just exactly as I thought, we should do it, but he should not.

"No, absolutely not, let him go AMA, we're not going to play his game, I don't care if his leg falls off, he'll probably die of lung cancer before that happens anyway." My sarcasm was, at that time, a little out of line. "Wait," I quickly backtracked. "Let me call my manager and ask her what she thinks."

I took a minute to dial my boss. I explained the situation and what I had already initiated, the AMA discussion, the social workers intervention and the request for twice a day trip outside to smoke. She, without any pondering, immediately agreed with me. We were not going to accommodate the smoking requests just to keep him in the hospital. He was an adult and he could make his own decisions. He would have to decide between smoking and medical treatment. I reiterated my conversation with Gary who went back to Randy's bed for the final discussion. After informing him that smoking was not an option, and if he wanted to leave the building to smoke, he would have to sign the AMA form, Randy simply said, "O.K. I'll think about it."

On that day, he chose to stay, but not before he made it clear that he was the one who would make the decision as to what he was going to do. He made sure the nurses knew that he knew that he had the right to make the choices. He wanted us all to know that he was in control of the decision that he made. On that day, many of the nurses were hoping that Randy would sign out AMA. They were hoping that he would go outside, have his cigarette and not come back. Every day if it wasn't the smoking debate, Randy was demanding other things. It was only a few hours after the smoking dispute was over, that Randy asked for a phone. There are no phones at the bedsides in the ICU. The patients are usually too sick to be answering phone calls, so phones are not one of the many items that must be at each bedside. We do have phones that we take to individual beds, plug into the wall and allow patients to make calls, and sometimes we will transfer important calls to the bedside of the more stable patients. When the call is finished, we once again, take the phone away.

Randy requested a phone; he didn't say who he was going to call. Some of us were hoping he would call a cab and go home. As he dialed the phone, he quietly mumbled that he was calling his sister. He spent some time talking, a short conversation that was quiet and calm. Whatever he called her for wasn't causing any outburst so we didn't really pay attention, there seemed to be no problem—we thought. But later that evening, his sister came to visit him. She brought two large boxes of Randy's belongings. Everything that had been in the shopping cart was now on the floor around his bed.

"No, no, no, this cannot stay here." I interrupted the delivery.

"I need my stuff," Randy objected. His sister, Bobbie, simply stood there and watched our interaction. Her eyes showed me she was not aware of the dynamics of the situation.

"There is not enough room for all of this to be in your small space," I continued to force the issue.

"I just brought his things like he asked me to do. I didn't realize it wasn't allowed," Bobbie started apologizing.

"It's O.K. you didn't do anything wrong," I tried to reassure her. "But you can see the problem we will have if you leave all this stuff," I wanted to say garbage "in this small space."

Randy continued to argue and push me to allow all his items to stay with him. We, once again, compromised. "You can look through the boxes and keep what will fit on this one bedside table. You cannot keep it all." And with that, I would not budge.

Randy and his sister sorted out the most important things for his survival. More videotapes, some socks, his favorite throw blanket and a few personal care items were some of the things that Randy felt he could not live without. His sister boxed up the rest and carried them out with her. On her way out, she apologized again. We had a short conversation and she told me that she and Randy had never gotten along well with each other. They had lead different lives, and Randy chose to live on the streets. Bobbie wanted to make sure I knew that she would be available to help Randy, but Randy would not be allowed to live with her. "I will keep his stuff for him and when he needs it I'll get it to him." And before she left she added, "If there is anything he needs, let me know." I assured her that we would be calling if we needed her and thanked her again for taking the clutter back to her garage.

As I returned to the unit, I saw that Randy was quickly setting up camp in the ICU. He was sorting his belonging and rearranging the tables and VCR around his bed. He was placing his most-used items on the foot of his bed. He was burrowing in for a lengthy stay!

He was demanding, rude, and often just a pain in the neck. When his meals would come, he would always request something different. If he had vanilla pudding on his tray, he would ask the nurse to call the kitchen and ask them to send butterscotch. If the nurse would refuse, he would act out, yelling and disturbing the entire unit. Each time his nurse would walk by his bed, he would request another item out of the refrigerator, ice cream, custard, soda, or crackers. During Randy's stay in ICU, he gained twenty pounds. All he did was sit and watch movies and order the nurses back and forth to the refrigerator. We continued to give him his antibiotics and tolerated his request in order to maintain peace in our unit.

Each day, the nurses had to take turns caring for Randy. Usually when a nurse has an assignment and she returns the following day, or even three days in a row, she will have the same assignment in order to maintain continuity. ICU nurses provide compassionate care to their critically ill patients every day. But to provide maid service to someone who is annoying and manipulative would quickly wear on your nerves, your compassion, and your patience. So with Randy, no one wanted to be his nurse for more that one day at a time.

After a few weeks, we scheduled a special care conference. This meeting included his physician, the discharge planner, the nursing manager, our medical director, and all the disciplines involved in his care. The medical director, who appreciates how hard the ICU nurses work, was trying to resolve this unfortunate situation. The physical needs of the patient as well as the psychological needs of the nurses needed to be addressed. Randy needed another two weeks of antibiotics in order for his physician to feel comfortable that the infection would be clear, and it would be safe for him to return to his unsanitary lifestyle. But the hostility that his demanding, controlling behavior was causing in the entire unit needed to be dealt with as well. The nurses felt that Randy was simply manipulating them in order to try to maintain control. After the conference it was decided that the nurses were not to give into Randy's excessive tedious demands and if he started escalating and making trouble, security would be called immediately. If Randy chose not to abide by the rules, he could leave the hospital.

* * *

Who are the homeless? There is no stereotype to describe the homeless. Most of them have lived what we consider "normal" lives at one time. Some have families; some have lost their jobs; some live on the streets because they have nowhere else, and some choose to live on the streets instead of living with family or friends who have opened their homes to them. Many of the homeless have physical illnesses, drug addictions and alcoholism, and multiple health problems. Many have mental illnesses, bipolar disease and schizophrenia. Some are veterans or victims of domestic violence. They are people, human beings who have, in the eyes of most, become a different class of people because of the poverty they live with daily. But these people were, at one time, just like you and me. The difference is that they don't have a house to curl up in every night. Many look daily for a warm place to spend the night, and often must sleep in a different place each night. Some return to the same place for solace. The winter is additionally hard for these people. To stay warm and to stay healthy is a challenge. They work daily to acquire their needs, food, shelter, and warmth. They work hard to maintain control of their life and every situation. They must stay in control of their situation, because in an instant their life's possessions, or even their life could be gone.

* * *

With the initiation of the new plan of care, Randy would not get everything he wanted, whenever he wanted. The nurses would be given more authority to say no to him, just as they would to their own children. And the security guards would be available to the nurses immediately for any problems. Randy was made aware of this new plan, and he begrudgingly accepted the new boundaries. The following few weeks were much more tolerable than the first weeks. Randy settled into a routine, breakfast followed by a movie, lunch, followed by a walk with physical therapy and a nap, then dinner and another movie. We encouraged him to increase the amount of food on his meal trays and he stopped nagging the nurses for additional food requests. Randy was given control of his meals and activities and the nurses were given control of their time. Peace was achieved once again in the ICU.

Finally, after Randy had completed his antibiotic treatment, it was time to be discharged. His physician came mid-morning, wrote the discharge orders and said "Get him out of here." The discharge planner was informed of the discharge order, and the nursing manager was also told.

We now had a plan. We would call Randy's sister; she would come pick him up and we would be rid of him. Randy was cooperating with this plan, but when he phoned his sister, she was not home. We waited, and called again and again and again, there was no answer. By the time Randy reached his sister, she was just about to go to work. She promised that she would come and pick him up after work, but that would not be until after dark. Randy did not want to wait; he wanted to be able to leave before it got dark. He was homeless; he needed to go to wherever he was going to sleep before dark. He needed to determine where that would be and he couldn't do that in the darkness of night.

Occasionally, we provide a taxi for patients who need a ride home when they don't have one. Homeless, poor, and others may need a taxi rather that wait until the next day for a friend or family to provide transportation. The cost of the taxi is considerably less than the cost of another night stay in the hospital. Randy wasn't going to have to stay another night, but to stay until nine in the evening wasn't a good option for him either. Because waiting until nine o'clock that evening for a ride would be a hardship for him, we initiated the request for a taxi. It wasn't that simple though. When we provide a taxi we have to put a specific address on the voucher. Randy had no address to go to, he had no home and no specific destination. He wanted to go to a corner market in the neighborhood near the field where he slept. The storeowner would allow him to panhandle in front of that market and get some cash. He needed to do this before dark and if he waited for Bobbie to pick him up, it would be too late.

However, there were more problems. The nurse manager did not want to discharge him to "nowhere." How could we send him to a market? How could we send him to a field? But that is where he wanted to go. That was his home. It may not be what most of us consider a home, but that is where Randy called home. Why would we impose our beliefs on him? Randy was willing to go home, but needed a ride. We could provide him with a ride, but wouldn't take him where he wanted to go.

All afternoon we struggled to make that discharge happen. Randy was ready to go and was waiting for a ride. But the decision to take him to nowhere was not easy. Several managers had to get involved including the nursing manager and the manager of the discharge planning. Each of them had to consult a variety of people to assure they were doing the right thing. The right thing is to take the patient where he wants to go. All he was asking for was a ride to a corner market about five miles from the hospital.

As the afternoon was getting late, Randy again began getting restless. How can we get him to where he needs to be? Randy was trying to be cooperative and our managers were standing in his way. By now, we had all come to know Randy. The last few weeks had been much more tolerable than the beginning of his stay, now all he wanted to do is go home and our bosses were dragging their feet.

At three o'clock Randy called me to his bedside. He inquired about the plan for his discharge. I explained to him that my boss was uncomfortable sending him to a corner market. I asked him if there was another place where he could go. "How about a hotel, close to the market," I suggested. "I'm sure my boss would prefer to deliver you to a hotel rather than a market or a field."

The closest hotel to that part of town was several miles away. A hotel was not an option. Randy stuck to his choice of where he wanted to go. He needed to go to that market.

"Is there anyone else who could pick you up? Any other way to get there?" I was trying to accommodate his needs.

He had no one, and no other ideas. But suddenly Randy came up with an alternative. "I ride the bus all the time. I know the bus schedules. I could ride the bus."

"There is a bus stop, just outside the door of the hospital. What bus line goes to your market?" Now I was finally moving toward discharge.

He gave me the number and informed me that the bus he needed had a connection at the commuter train station that was a short distance from the hospital. He could catch the bus outside the hospital and transfer at the commuter train station.

"But I don't want to sign out AMA," Randy shared with me.

"You will not be going AMA, you have officially been discharged, you can walk out of here any time you want." With that explanation, Randy seemed relieved that he was no longer creating problems for the nurses in the ICU.

Now we had a plan, Randy and I. He would wait until four in the evening for a taxi voucher. If the managers were not going to provide a taxi ride by four o'clock, he would take the bus. That would get him to where he needed to go and he would be there before dark.

By making the bus plans, I felt I had gone against the wishes of the administration. But at that time, I needed to do what was right for the patient. Taking the bus and getting to where he needed to go was a better choice than waiting for a taxi or waiting for his sister and not being able to accomplish what he knew had to be done before twilight. Randy was content that we were working together as a team. I was trying to accommodate his unique life style and not imposing my own beliefs on him.

At three-thirty, I received word that the taxi voucher would be approved and, despite the objections of the manager, Randy could go to his corner market of choice. We spent the next thirty minutes packing his belongings into plastic bags. We gave him his cigarette lighter back from the safe holding place and put it with his precious cigarettes. He packed a few newspapers and a few other items, but wanted to leave his jacket. He didn't want to take it because it took up too much room. "I don't have enough space for it," he objected.

I suddenly turned into a mother and insisted he take the jacket. "You need the jacket, it's going to get cold when the sun goes down."

In addition to insisting on the jacket, we gave him a few crackers and sodas from the refrigerator, just in case he got hungry. The rest of his belongings were bagged and left in a safe place. Bobbie would come pick them up after work.

We called the taxi and when it arrived, Randy walked out to the lobby. We all said good-bye and good-luck, meaning it, but really wanting to say, "please don't come back" as he climbed into the back seat of his ride.

* * *

Randy taught us a few things. The homeless live a hard life, and they need to be tough to survive. On the surface, they are annoying, ungrateful, and obnoxious, like Randy was in the beginning. The shell had to be tough for survival. But inside, they are ordinary people and just want to do what is right for themselves. Each of these homeless people has learned, through trial and error, what is best for their own survival. They have learned how to survive on the streets, and if it requires a taxi to nowhere, that is what we need to do for them. Those of us, who live in the comforts of our warm houses, must accommodate their needs. We cannot impose our beliefs on them; we must help them to achieve what it takes to be successful and endure.

Since caring for Randy, and a few others, I have developed a different opinion of the homeless I often see walking the streets. I used to think they were all "crazy" or "drug addicts." But now I know these are real people. They are real people who, for some reason, are down on their luck; real people who have no other choice, and real people who sometimes choose to live out in the open. We cannot assume that because we think they need to be someplace, we should take them there. Sometimes the best place for them is no-where.

It Takes a Certain Kind of Person

One day I received word that a patient was being transferred into ICU from the floor. He had been admitted the previous day with a diagnosis of a GI bleed. At this time, no one had determined if the gastrointestinal bleeding originated from the stomach, small intestines, large intestines, or the colon. But he was having bloody stools and his blood count was going down. Just before his transfer to ICU, as he was being prepared for the journey downstairs, he decided he must first visit the lavatory. He needed one last stop before his journey to the ICU. On his way to the lavatory, he suddenly felt faint; he fell to the floor and lost control of his bowels. As he lay in a pool of fresh blood mixed with stool, momentarily unconscious, his nurse called a Code Blue. The Code Blue activated the emergency team who would help in this situation. The code team found the patient on the floor, awake and alert, but pale and diaphoretic. He was more embarrassed than he was hurt. The team, now aware that they were not needed to do CPR or resuscitate this patient, quickly applied gloves, scooped the patient up off the floor onto the gurney and rushed him to his awaiting bed in the ICU.

As I received the patient, my first concern was for his safety and what needed to be done to stabilize him. We hooked him up to monitors, and started infusing an IV at a rapid rate, and called his doctor. My next thoughts moved toward, *how am I going to clean up this mess?* He was covered with bloody stool from the waist down. His gown, his boxer shorts, and all the linens were soaked with a foul smelling blood and stool mixture. Once he was stable, he needed to be cleaned. Two of us gathered a clean set of linens, extra washcloths and towels and went to work. Removing layers of linens and layers of clothing, we stripped him naked and went to work.

As we cleaned this needy patient of his embarrassing mess, he continually apologized for making us perform this nasty task. We reassured him that there was no need to apologize for an event that he could not control. We assured him that we do this, and many other tasks that are even nastier, all the time. We joked with him, in an effort to make him feel better, that we like this kind of stuff, that's why we are nurses.

As I was cleaning this disgusting mess from all the crevasses, I wondered who else would do this kind of work. I do get paid good money, but not everyone would do this, no matter how much they got paid. As I have said several times before, it takes a certain kind of person to be a nurse. Not everyone can do this kind of work.

When discussing this same topic later that day, one of my co-workers said, "Prostitutes get paid a lot of money too, but not everyone can do that kind of work either."

CHAPTER 11

To Say or Not to Say

When the nurse is asked, "Please don't let my mom die."
What is she to say?

As I've said many times, the ICU is reserved for patients who are sicker than most. Because of this, the family members will often be more concerned, more worried, and more anxious than others. They ask many questions, look for answers, and search for reassurance in many different ways.

Often the stress that the family members are experiencing will result in a considerable number of questions and requests. Sometimes these requests may seem unrealistic. Most often the family is just trying to reassure themselves.

We may not be able to grant all the requests, but it's not unrealistic that we take the time to answer all the questions so the relatives receive the appropriate information and the reassurance they are seeking.

Because of the increased anxiety the family will grasp at any and every word spoken. Often they will focus on one comment. They will fixate on one word they hear. They will sometimes ask for reassurance we cannot give.

A wife asks the nurse, "How's he doing?"

The nurse responds casually, "He's doing fine."

This is because, to the nurse, "fine" may mean that his low blood pressure is responding to the medications and he hasn't had any life-threatening arrhythmias on her shift.

The wife holds onto the "he's doing *fine*" and goes home to get some rest.

Later that evening her husband suddenly has a cardiac arrest. That wife will repeat over and over, "She said he was fine, I just don't understand."

Likewise, when a husband pleads to the nurse and says, "Please don't let my wife die," the nurse cannot assure him she won't let her die. If an unexpected event occurs in the middle of the night, the nurse has failed the husband by promising something she cannot control.

I learned early in my career not to make promises, not to say anything that cannot be guaranteed, and not to promise anything that I do not have control over.

* * *

Elsie came to the ICU after experiencing the sudden onset of an excruciating headache. After the CT scan confirmed blood in the brain, her physician admitted her to the ICU. Blood is not normally in the tissues of the brain, but should remain within the vascular system. When a cerebral blood vessel leaks, blood spills out into the brain tissue. The skull, a hard bone, does not provide an area for expansion within the head. There is normally just enough space for the brain, the blood vessels and the cerebral spinal fluid. An increase in any one of those three space-consuming components will cause an increase in intracranial pressure, resulting in a severe headache.

Elsie—like all unstable neuro patients—required ICU care because of the risk that her condition could change drastically within minutes. Neuro patients require frequent assessments, which include: monitoring their level of consciousness; assuring they are awake; confirming they are oriented to person, place and time, and they are able to follow commands. In addition, neuro assessments include monitoring the pupils for changes. Pupils normally respond equally to light. When light is shone into the eyes, both pupils will constrict in reaction to the bright light. If one pupil does not respond briskly and equally to the other, increased intra cranial pressure is suspected. All patients with a diagnosis of intra cranial bleeding are monitored closely and assessed frequently for changes.

Elsie was a 28-year-old woman, married with a three-year-old daughter. During her ten days in the ICU, tests and scans located the position of the cerebral aneurism that had caused the bleeding in her brain. An aneurism is an abnormal ballooning of a blood vessel. The ballooning caused a weakening of the vessel, and when the weakened wall leaked, blood spilled out into the brain cavity. Luckily for Elsie, the bleeding stopped spontaneously without significant damage. Sometimes, for those who are not as lucky, the bleeding will not stop and massive stroke or death occurs. Now that Elsie was safe in our ICU, we monitored her closely, watching for signs of re-bleeding, while waiting for any spasms of the irritated blood vessel to resolve. After she was stable, the neuro surgeon would take her to surgery and repair the aneurysm.

Because Elsie was so close to my age, we developed a close relationship, one different from my normal attachment to many of my patients. Each day I would care for her, watch her closely, and assure her that everything would be just fine. Each day her husband, Ben, would sneak her daughter into the unit, breaking the rules that no one under the age of fourteen was allowed to visit. Shannon would sit quietly on mama's lap and share her laughter and happiness. Ben and Elsie could not share their worries with their beautiful daughter. Shannon only knew that mama was sick and needed to have the doctors fix the bruise in her brain.

We monitored, we assessed, and we waited until it was safe for Elsie to have the brain surgery. She waited patiently, showing no signs of complications. We limited her activities, we avoided stress, and we watched her closely. During her stay in ICU, she sat patiently and waited until the time would come when the surgeon could resolve the problem that caused this sudden threat to her life.

The time had finally come. There were no more spasms of her cerebral blood vessels, so surgery was scheduled. Elsie would have her head shaved and the aneurysm repaired.

"Let's get it done, so I can go home," I remember her saying when she was told the surgery would take place within a few days. But the day before the surgery, Elsie was visibly worried. She asked all the appropriate questions while Ben was there to hear the answers.

"How long will the surgery take? What will they do with my hair? How long will I be in the hospital?" All expected questions for a young mother facing brain surgery. She was aware of all the risks of the surgery, re-bleeding, stroke, and even death. But the risks of not having the surgery were far greater than the risk of any untoward effects of the surgery. She could not risk not having the surgery and perhaps some day suffering a sudden death from the bursting of that same aneurysm.

As Elsie was preparing for her trip to the operating room, we once again sneaked Shannon into the unit. This time, we were not as discreet. Shannon sat proudly on mama's bed, kissing her as she was pushed out of the unit. As we left the unit and passed by the waiting room, it was time for Shannon to disembark the rolling bed she had been enjoying with her mom. Ben and Shannon gave Elsie one last kiss as she was pushed toward the operating suite. As Elsie was saying her good-byes to her family, she looked up at me, with pleading eyes and said, "I'm scared."

I impulsively answered her concern with what I felt was the only possible answer. "Don't worry, everything will be fine. You have a great doctor and you'll be fine." I told her what I felt in my heart. I knew she would be just fine, she was young and she was in the excellent hands of a great neuro-surgeon. "I'll be here when you get back," I assured her.

As the tears collected in her eyes, the orderly continued to roll her away from Ben and Shannon.

It was hours later, more than the expected time allotment, when Elsie finally returned to the ICU. The surgeon accompanied her as she was wheeled back into the unit. He sat at the foot of the bed as we reestablished all of the monitoring devices she had left behind, in addition to some newly acquired tubes and infusions that had been initiated during surgery. Elsie was on a ventilator, supporting her life. This, most likely would be weaned off when the anesthesia wore off, and Elsie woke up. But, the look on the neuro-surgeon's face told me this might not be so. The look on his face was not the usual happy expression we always saw from this surgeon. His eyes were saddened—he was not speaking. He waited until we settled Elsie back into her abandoned ICU bed before he shared the dreadful experience of the operating room.

He explained that as soon as he located the aneurysm, and moved the brain tissue away, it blew again. Simply by releasing the natural pressure, which the brain was holding on the weakened artery, allowed the bleeding to resume. The weakened vessel exploded in his fingers. With the excessive amount of blood, he could not control the bleeding.

Elsie's aneurysm had ruptured before the talented hands could prevent death. The surgeon suspected that Elsie had sustained massive brain injury due to the bleeding and the swelling of the brain. The prognosis was poor, only time would tell. I suddenly realized that Elsie may not be "just fine" as I had promised.

Ben was allowed into the room as soon as we stabilized Elsie. He had already been informed of the events and was visibly shaken. Shannon had gone home with her grandmother, sheltered from the crisis that was unfolding around her mother. Now, all we could do was wait, wait and see if a miracle would happen, wait and see if Elsie would wake up, wait and see how the events would play out.

I stayed close to Ben as I finished my shift. I explained all of the new monitoring devices, what the next nurse would be watching for, and answered all of his questions as candidly as I could. As I was leaving for the evening, I assured him that the night shift nurse would do everything she could for his wife. I contracted with him to try to get some sleep, in the waiting room, and the nurse would come wake him if any changes occurred. And finally, I reminded him that I would be back in the morning.

When I came back in the morning, I met with an unshaven, half-sleepy devoted husband who had not left the bedside all night. After listening to report, and upon assessing my only patient, it was evident that Elsie was "brain dead." Her pupils were dilated and not responding to the bright flashlight that was so often shone into her eyes. No reflexes were present, no gag, no cough, and no blink. The bleeding and the swelling had caused so much brain damage that there was no brain function left. The only thing left was to confirm with an EEG—which, by noon, told us that there were no brain waves present in this young wife and mother.

The events of the next twenty-four hours were devastating. The family was provided time to realize Elsie was dead inside that otherwise healthy body. Ben made the decision to donate all of Elsie's organs that could be used to save the lives of others. We worked together with the Donor Network, assuring that Ben's needs were met. But, his only need was to have his wife back, and we couldn't provide that. He was strong, as any husband and father could be. He made all the arrangements, said his good-bye, and left his wife in the hands of the transplant team.

Ben stayed long enough to say thank you to all the nurses. He truly appreciated the excellent care his wife received. He especially appreciated those who broke the rules to allow his precious daughter to spend time with her mother during what we now knew were her last days. He understood that we all did everything we could to save the life of his wife. Ben now had to go home and explain to his daughter that mama would not be coming home from the hospital—despite the fact the nurse told her "everything would be fine."

* * *

I remember Elsie, Ben, and Shannon, and I remember that I was confident when I told them that she would be fine. I assured all of them that everything would be OK. I still today, feel guilty for providing them with what might have been false reassurance. And now, in my current practice, I have learned not to promise, and not to give assurances for things I cannot guarantee.

Family members are always looking for reassurance that their loved one will get better. They want security that the patient will improve, that nothing bad will happen. But, I've found, more than with Elsie, that the nurse cannot make those promises. We cannot guarantee that each of our critically ill, and often unstable patients will not die.

The comforting nature of most nurses makes it difficult not to be able to assure the patient or family that everything will be fine. But, the truth is, we can't control the uncertain outcomes of many of our clients, so we must provide the reassurance they are looking for without promises.

I frequently get asked, "Is she going to make it?" I always hope so. But I never say, "of course she is." Instead, I respond with the truth. "We're doing everything we can" or "we're trying very hard" and I go on to explain all of the treatments and interventions we are doing in order to allow that patient to "make it."

Sometimes the family asks, "Is he going to die?" Yet another question that is too hard to answer. So, I never say, "no, he's not." Instead, I reply, "I hope not, I'm doing everything I can to help him and get him better." I follow that type of comment with more explanations of the care I am providing and what I am doing to keep the patient from dying. Often what is really behind these types of questions is simply a request for more information and the reassurance that their family member is receiving the best care possible. I have learned, never make promises; never guarantee what I cannot provide.

Elsie was looking to me for reassurance. I hope I gave her what she needed. I hope my last words to her were comforting. But since then, I've learned not to make promises. I've learned some things are left better unsaid. Reassurances without promises, that's what the nurse must provide. I have learned what to say and what not to say.

CHAPTER 12

Do Not Resuscitate—Please

When do we stop inflicting pain and suffering on our
patients who have no chance for survival?

"Code Blue" is the announcement heard when there is a medical emergency. CPR is started; a life is saved. But what if one doesn't want CPR? What if one doesn't want to be resuscitated? What do we do then? We, the healthcare team, consult with the patient and the family in order to provide the care they want. Sometimes, CPR is not the best intervention. Patients, who have been suffering with long chronic illnesses, may choose not to have their life prolonged. Patients, who are old and have lived a long independent life, may not want to live if they cannot go home to their previous level of independence. These patients may have had discussions with their family. They may have made decisions that, when the time comes, don't prolong their life. In this situation, the doctor will write a DNR order. DNR means Do Not Resuscitate. To the healthcare providers, this means if the heart stops, or the patient stops breathing, the nurses will provide comfort care and not delay the inevitable.

Sometimes it is unfortunate that these discussions do not happen before they are needed. Sometimes it's not until the patient actually stops breathing, or when the patient's heart stops that we, the healthcare providers, start CPR and then have the conversation with the family to determine if this is in fact what the patient wanted us to do.

* * *

Ronald was an 87-year-old man who came to our ICU from the medical unit. Ronald was admitted to the hospital a week prior with abdominal pain. The doctors had done several tests to determine the cause of Ronald's pain. X-rays and gastrointestinal studies were thus far inconclusive. After a week of tests and observation, Ronald started experiencing difficulty breathing. I received a call from the medical floor charge nurse informing me that he was going to be transferred to our unit. We were also receiving another patient from a different unit at the same time. Unfortunately we only had one empty bed. The charge nurse on Ronald's floor assured me he was relatively stable. "He is short of breath but we just gave him a mild sedative and he seems much better." And, she suggested I take the other patient first and call when the next bed was available.

Within an hour, we transferred a patient out of ICU, prepared the room, and accepted Ronald to the only empty bed. As we moved him from the gurney to the bed, I immediately started performing my physical exam. Even before I placed my stethoscope to Ronald's chest, I could see that his respiratory status was in jeopardy. His breathing was very rapid; forty times a minute, and shallow. His color was pale so I made sure his oxygen was connected to the regulator promptly. Three liters of oxygen may not be enough for him, even though the small finger monitor told me his oxygen saturation was reading 98%. His wide eyes looked directly into my face. It was as if I could see right through them to see that he was scared. His wandering glances seemed to be searching his new surroundings for signs he would receive the help he desperately needed.

His lungs were clear; his cardiac monitor showed a rapid heart rate of about 110 beats per minute and he had no significant edema. The rest of my assessment was unremarkable. However, my gut was telling me Ronald's condition was not unremarkable, and he was not fine like the medical charge nurse reported earlier. With a respiratory rate in the forties, pale skin and the scared look in his eyes, I could see he was not fine.

My first call was to the respiratory therapist. "Come to ICU 5, I need reinforcements, and on your way find out what Ronald's ABG results were." I glanced in the chart to see if we had an order for a respiratory treatment—nothing ordered. Within minutes, the respiratory therapist was beside me with the ABG results. Ronald's oxygen level was 75—lower than normal; his carbon dioxide level was also low, 27. This told me that he was ventilating fine, blowing off his carbon dioxide, but he was not getting enough oxygen. I considered increasing the oxygen dose, maybe use a mask, but as I pondered my options, I watched Ronald breath faster and faster, he was struggling to breath.

Forget the increase in oxygen, we need bi-pap. The respiratory therapist set up the machine while I called the pulmonologist to get the order. The bi-pap mask, with supplemental oxygen, would push extra oxygen into his lungs each time he took a breath.

About that time, his wife and daughter came into the room. I explained to them what we were doing and how the bi-pap mask would help Ronald. The daughter asked me how long this mask would take to help her father. She could see that he was in distress just as I could. I couldn't answer her question, but I could explain to both of them that we were going to try this method and see what happened.

It didn't take long to see that the bi-pap was not helping Ronald. We were supplementing his oxygen and his breathing efforts, but his respiratory rate was increasing. Now the monitor showed me a respiratory rate in the fifties. I made another call to the pulmonologist and told him the current treatment was not working. Despite the fact that the oxygen saturation says Ronald was getting enough oxygen, his respiratory rate was increasing. "I think you need to come, he's going to tire out." This was my way of suggesting that poor Ronald needed to be intubated, the breathing tube inserted to his lungs, and placed on a ventilator.

Within minutes, the pulmonologist arrived at the bedside. We explained to the wife and daughter what we were going to do. "He's not breathing well, and the bi-pap is not helping him as fast as we need it to. What we need to do now is to put a tube in his throat and attach it to a machine that will help him breath." After a brief pause I continued, "Is that what you want?" I always try to ask this question before we intubate. Maybe there has been some discussion and this was not what Ronald would want.

The daughter shook her head very rapidly, giving us permission to proceed as she wrapped her arm around her mother and they turned to leave the room. I asked her and her mother to step into the waiting room and give us a few minutes. I assured them that I would call them back in when we were done. The daughter took a minute before leaving and told her dad we were going to put a tube in his throat and it would help him breath. But at that moment, he didn't seem to acknowledge her words.

The team, including the doctor, the respiratory therapist, and myself, went into action. As we were performing our life-saving interventions for this now pale, distressed 87-year-old man, the pulmonologist told us this same man was in his office just a few years ago. He had all the office gals laughing with his jokes. "Some character" he was, "a very funny guy." But what we were seeing now was not a funny guy; he was in a lot of trouble. Following some mild sedation, we intubated Ronald and placed him on a ventilator so he could relax. The machine would breath for him; his work was over for now.

I asked the pulmonologist what he thought was happening to Ronald. Was it lung disease, pneumonia, or what? His response was simply "old age."

As I looked around the room and saw all the too familiar machines attached to Ronald, I respond, "I guess you can't die of old age any more."

"Not in the hospital, you can't. We put you on machines first," and he wrote the orders for the interventions that we had just completed.

Ronald seemed to be stable on the ventilator; the sedation was keeping him relaxed. The ventilator was helping to relieve his work of breathing. And his family was calmly sitting by his bed. That didn't last long, despite our efforts. Ronald had different ideas about what he was going to do. Ronald decided he wasn't willing to live any more and his heart rate started dropping. Sixty—fifty—forty—thirty beats per minute. As I reached for the ambu bag to manually force air into Ronald's lungs, and pushed the Code Blue button, another ICU nurse descended on my bedside. She calmly asked the family to leave the room, "Please wait in the waiting room," she commanded.

"Code Blue ICU, Code Blue ICU, Code Blue ICU" rang through the entire hospital. The emergency room doctor who responded to our code was much like the young "Doogie Houser." He looked about fifteen-years-old—he could have been one of my own sons. Despite the fact that he was barely half my age, it was his job to run the code now.

The code team arrived, we did CPR, gave medications, started more IV fluids, and Ronald just kept getting bluer and bluer. No heart beat, no sign of life. Two other ICU nurses were helping with this code, so I excused myself from the room after informing them I was going to talk to the family. We had left them unattended long enough. I went to the waiting room, and the family was calmly watching television. It seemed that they had no clue their dad was dying on the other side of the wall. Now the grandson had joined his mother and his grandmother. The word was out that grandpa was not doing well.

I squatted down in front of the daughter, who had emerged as the decision maker, and told her that we were continuing to do CPR on her dad. I explained, once again, what happened and that the team was doing chest compressions, giving medications, and infusing fluids for the entire time they had been waiting here in the waiting room. Suddenly the realization came over all of their faces. I felt like I needed to ask, "Is this what you want us to do?"

"Is he on life support?" she inquired.

"Yes, the ventilator we put him on earlier is life support." I answered that basic question, and then proceeded with more as I looked into her wide eyes, trying to understand what was moving rapidly through her mind. "Right now, we are doing chest compressions and giving him medications to try to get his heart going again."

Questions came flowing like a levy had just broken. "Will he make it?" "Will he be able to go home and garden again?" "What will he be like if he does make it?" "Have you seen 87-year-old men survive this?" "If he does survive, do you think he will need to live in a nursing home?" All of which are very appropriate questions.

I answered the questions the best I could. I kept repeating, "from my nursing opinion," because I didn't want them to think that I was giving them medical advice. They needed answers in order to make a decision, but too many of their questions were answered with my sympathetic "I don't know."

After a few moments, Ronald's daughter spoke up and said, "He wouldn't want to live on machines."

Then his wife added, "We have talked about this." Following a short pause, she continued, "He doesn't want to be on life support." Another pause …"if he can't be in his garden, he won't be happy."

After a moment to absorb this newly expressed information, I asked if they had shared this information with his physician.

"We didn't think he was that sick," she whispered, as she wiped tears from her cheeks.

They didn't think he was that sick. How sick do you need to be, to discuss your end-of-life choices with your doctor? How sick do you have to be, to tell the hospital staff, when you are admitted to the hospital, that you do not want life support? Why don't people talk about these things and discuss them with their doctors before they are in this dreadful situation? All these were questions I couldn't answer then, and today I'm still struggling with the same dilemma.

When I was taking care of Ronald, it wasn't the norm for every patient to be asked about health care directives on admission. It wasn't addressed as a routine question like allergies, medications and medical history, like it is in more recent years.

As I was contemplating what I was going to do with this newfound information, the daughter interrupted my thoughts with a question, the same question that I was already pondering.

"What are we going to do now?"

Before I had a chance to try to explain what we could do now, she started crying.

The few moments I gave her to gather her composure seemed like an eternity of silence. Finally, Ronald's daughter spoke up and said, "He wouldn't want to be on machines."

Her mother sat silently by her side with wet, pleading eyes.

Once again, in the silence of my own mind, I kept repeating the questions. *Why didn't someone make Ronald's wishes known to those of us who have been taking care of him for the past week? Why hadn't Ronald told his doctor, so it could be on his medical record? What was I going to do now?*

She looked at her mother, and then back to me. As she shook her head side to side, in a crackling voice she requested, "Oh God. Can we just let him be?"

I tried to use gentle words, even though my head was screaming with my own questions. *Why didn't you say something earlier? Why didn't you tell the doctor? Why did you wait until this 87-year-old man is in cardiac arrest to share this vital information?* But, I couldn't say this to the family in this very delicate time of distress.

"It looks like you guys all agree that your dad would not want this." I gave them a questioning look that elicited simultaneous nods of agreement.

I had to repeat what I thought they wanted. "Do you want me to go in there and tell them to stop?" Each of them nodded approval. They didn't want to, but they each knew they had to, because that was what Ronald would want.

I tried to give the daughter a comforting touch as I stood up from my squatting position. "I'll be right back" I assured them. Then I turned and went back into the ICU.

Still no pulse, CPR in progress, the code team was still at work. As I approached the bed, I told the young emergency room doctor that I had just been talking to the family, the wife, the daughter, and the grandson, and they wanted us to stop what we were doing and let him go peacefully.

I informed him that they had told me that he would not want this and they wanted us to stop.

The young doctor "Houser" turned toward those surrounding the patient in the bed and said, "Continue CPR."

I immediately responded, "The family wants us to stop." I'm sure my eyes were as wide as silver dollars. I couldn't believe he would blatantly go against the family wishes.

"I'll talk to them," he said as he brushed by me and headed to the waiting area.

I couldn't believe he wouldn't believe me. But if he needed to hear for himself, fine. I'm sure they'll tell him the same as they told me.

I followed him back to the waiting area, where now the grand-daughter had joined the rest of the family. There were four of them. Young doctor "Houser" reiterated to the family everything I had just told them. He explained that Ronald had received several rounds of resuscitative medications, which had failed to restart his heart. He explained that the code team was still working to bring him back.

"I understand that you might want us to do something differ-ent." Now they were all looking puzzled. *What kind of question was that? What was he talking about?* I was puzzled now too. *Why didn't he just say, do you want us to stop the code? Do you want us to let him pass away peacefully? Because that was what they wanted, they didn't want us to do something different, they wanted us to do nothing, noth-ing, leave Ronald alone.*

I suddenly realized that end-of-life discussions are not easy to initiate. I now realized that experience and comfort play a major role in these discussions. Despite what I thought was a vague question, the family was able to express their wishes to the doctor and he agreed to stop the code. As he turned to walk away, I again assured the family that I would be back soon and I would bring them all in the room to see Ronald.

As soon as I entered Ronald's room, just feet behind the doctor, we were informed that, believe it or not, Ronald now had a pulse. A weak pulse, but it was present. Despite the medication that was infusing to support his blood pressure, that too was barely present.

Now we had done exactly what Ronald had not wanted us to do. We kept him alive with life support measures. We had done this, because no one had expressed his wishes to his healthcare providers. Ronald's life was being supported now, whether he wanted it or not. We had already done all the emergency measures that would save his life; before the family told us the secret they seemed to be keeping from those very people who needed to know it. His breathing was supported by the ventilator, and his heart was supported by the multiple medications that were now infusing so precisely through the IV pumps.

What do we do now? We wait and see what happens. Maybe the weak pulse and blood pressure was due to the excessive amounts of resuscitation medication that were given when he was pulseless. Let's bring the family in, let them be with him, let them hold his hand, and wait for his heart to slow once again.

I returned to the waiting room to escort the family to the bedside. I wanted them to be with him while they could. I am a strong believer that the family should be at the bedside when the patient is dying. Even if we are coding the patient, the family can be there if they choose. This allows them to see that the healthcare team does truly do everything possible to save the life of the person they love.

After providing a few minutes of support to the family, I left them to be alone with their father, grandfather, husband. I wasn't sure how long the medication would continue to support the heart of this now pale, diaphoretic, lifeless body. I wanted them to spend the last moments with him. A few moments, because that is how long I was hoping that Ronald would have to endure all the interventions that he didn't want in the first place.

Before Dr. Houser left the unit, to return to his busy emergency department, I reminded him to write the DNR order. But he wasn't as eager as I was. As he left the unit, he looked directly at my shocked face and said, "Call the pulmonologist and have him talk to the family about a DNR, I'm not going to write that order, his own doctor needs to."

I stood paralyzed with shock! I couldn't believe he wasn't going to write the order. What was he thinking? What was he doing? I could only look at his age, his experience, and his comfort level with end-of-life issues, to understand where he was coming from.

I couldn't get to the phone fast enough. Another nurse collected some chairs for the family to gather supportingly around the bed. Unfortunately, my frustration was not alleviated when I spoke to the pulmonologist on the phone. He sympathetically told me that because he was simply a consulting doctor, he did not feel comfortable giving me an order for DNR. I was instructed to call the primary physician. He knew this patient better than the consulting pulmonologist and he should be the one to discuss this with the family and give that order.

One more phone call. I was going to make sure we did not torture Ronald any more. If he could not go back to his garden, he did not want to be kept alive. I spoke to the physician who was on call for Ronald's primary care doctor. He relayed that he did not feel comfortable making this decision and would not give me a verbal order. Didn't he know? The family had already made the decision. I was simply asking him to speak with the family and give me the DNR order. He was not going to accommodate Ronald's wishes or mine. He did agree to call Ronald's primary physician, discuss the issue with him and call me back.

Good! This was a glimmer of hope. Maybe now we could honor the family's wishes. Even though it was too late, we could prevent any more unwanted interventions. It seemed like an eternity, as we waited for the return call. We continued to adjust the Dopamine and Levophed infusions, which supported his weakened blood pressure. The blood pressure was 90/50 and the heart rate was 100 beats per minute. The patient was stable now, but I still worried that his old heart would give out again and we would once again have to start life-saving procedures … unless we had a DNR order from the physician.

I spent some more time with the family, updating them on what each of the medications were doing, and answering all of their questions and concerns. As I left the room, I was alerted that the primary physician was on the phone. I filled him in on what had happened to his patient of almost forty years. I explained that after the Code Blue, the family had shared with me that they had had discussions about life support, and Ronald had told them, when it was his time, he didn't want to be kept alive on machines. He sounded as frustrated as I was when hearing this for the first time. He asked me why they hadn't told him this earlier. I couldn't answer that question any better than I could answer many of the questions the family had been asking me all evening. After a complete update on Ronald's condition, I brought the daughter and the wife to the phone to speak to the doctor.

After a long discussion on the phone with the daughter, and then with the wife, I was once again speaking to the doctor. Our follow up conversation included sharing our combined frustration that all of this could have been prevented if this issue had been discussed and expressed before this emergency had happened. It was too late now; we had already prolonged death for a man who seemingly didn't want to have to go through what he was going through now. The primary doctor gave me the orders I needed over the phone. The orders that he wished he had known were needed before inflicting unnecessary pain and suffering to his long-time patient and friend. Because the family was worried that Ronald would suffer more if we removed the breathing tube, we decided to leave the ventilator in place. We would, however, start weaning down the support medications and if his old, weakened heart failed, we would allow it to stop. This time we had a DNR order that would allow Ronald's heart to stop when it could not go on any longer.

More family members were gathering now. The word had gotten out that the patriarch of the family was going to die and everyone needed to say their good-byes. Family members took turns sitting by the bedside, waiting; waiting for whatever was going to happen next.

As they asked me what to expect, I couldn't give them specifics. All I could do was give possibilities. It had been several hours since we kick-started his heart away from death. Now it seemed that his heart was thriving, despite the fact that we had lowered the dosages of the supportive medications. As we continued to wean the drips, his blood pressure showed us, he needed no support. I explained what the plan of care was. As we removed the medications that seemed to be supporting his vital signs, Ronald's blood pressure may start a slow deceleration. After the blood pressure, the heart rate may slowly deteriorate. I reassured them that we would provide him with medication to keep him comfortable, and when his heart stopped, we would not do CPR. We would let him pass peacefully. Everyone was finally in agreement with the same plan for compassionate comfort care. I encouraged them to stay at the bedside and when the time came, they could be there with him, as he leaves them for the last time.

The family started their all night vigil at the bedside. No one was going to leave Ronald alone. Each of them took turns sitting in the small hard chair next to his mattress while the others tried to catch brief naps in the waiting room. The entire family spent the night waiting for what they thought would come. But what we all expected to happen didn't happen that night, and, it didn't happen for several days.

Seven long days, the family kept their vigil. The medications had been stopped. The tests and interventions had been stopped. Everything had been stopped except the ventilator support. The machine that Ronald didn't want in the first place was still keeping him alive for seven long, lingering days. His family couldn't bear to remove the life support once it had been started, so Ronald, at 87-years-old, was kept alive with machines.

Seven long days, we turned, suctioned, bathed, and comforted this old man who never regained consciousness. We cared for him as we would any other ailing gentleman who might wake up. But mostly we provided gentle comfort for the family as they grieved through this lingering death, a prolonged death that could have been avoided.

Finally, at the end of the last day, as the sun was going down, Ronald's heart decided it was time for his last sunset. As the sun lowered over the horizon, so too did his weakened heart. As his family stood and watched, his heart was tiring out. His heart rate began to drop. Once again his pulse was slowing, seventy—sixty—fifty—forty. The time was near, he was tired and so was his heart. His breathing was desperate, against the assistance of the machine. As his blood pressure slowly deteriorated, his heart rate continued to follow. Slowly and calmly Ronald passed away; finally, without any further delays, with his family by his side.

In the end, Ronald was allowed to die peacefully. But not before he had to suffer through the torturous Code Blue, and then again, hanging onto life, so delicately throughout those last days. In the end, Ronald was allowed to die. But it was not how he wanted to go. He had discussions with his family, but no one told those who needed to know. Perhaps if someone, anyone had spoken about this before it was too late, Ronald would not have had to stay attached to that machine. Perhaps if Ronald and his family had discussed end-of-life options with his doctor, and again with the health care providers in the hospital, he would not have had to endure the long days and nights clinging to life support machines that he didn't want to be attached to in the first place.

* * *

During my frequent communications with Ronald's family, one of the questions his daughter asked me was, "What would you do if he was your dad?" I told her that I had had many, many discussions with both my parents. And that I understood how hard it was for her to make the decision, but in the end, we must remember the wishes of our parents. I understand because I have been in that position, and had to make a similar decision for my mom, and I know how hard it is.

My own mother has had many conversations with me about her own DNR status. Mom has Scleroderma, a chronic disease that results in hardening of the connective tissues. Mom suffers from congestive heart failure, and pulmonary fibrosis. She has lived for many years in pain and discomfort, but she will never be a burden to anyone. She has made her wishes known that she does not want to be on life support. Because of her pulmonary fibrosis, it is probably unrealistic to think that my mom would ever be weaned off a ventilator, once initiated. And she has made it known that she doesn't want to suffer on machines when her time comes.

Dad supports Mom's decision, as hard as it is for him. He knows Mom doesn't want to burden anyone and would not be happy living day after day connected to a machine. Because I am the only nurse in the family, I have been named as the durable power of attorney for healthcare for both of my parents. I will have to be the strong one to say no when the time comes, Dad will not be able to make that decision after over fifty years together. I anticipate making the decision for him, but we will do it together because that is what Mom wants. Just as Ronald's family did for their dad, we will do for our mom.

It's easy to sit on a couch or at a dinner table and discuss end-of-life issues. It's important for families to let each other know what they want. But when it comes time to actually tell the doctors to stop treatment, or even not to initiate that treatment, that is the hardest moment in anyone's life.

* * *

A few years ago my mom was admitted to the hospital with an acute episode of ulcerative colitis. The insides of her intestines were bleeding and sloughing off. The doctor informed us that surgery was the treatment of choice for this life-threatening ailment. However, because of my mother's underlying health disorders, she most likely would not survive surgery without having to be placed on a ventilator. Because of her chronic lung problem, once on a ventilator, it was highly likely that mom would not be able to be weaned off of ventilator support. Since Mom feels strongly about never initiating ventilator support, surgery was reluctantly ruled out as an option. As the emergency room physician was reviewing mom's chart, he noted that she had a DNR order from a previous admission. The doctor looked across the gurney at me and initiated that dreaded discussion about rewriting the order for this admission. My mom and my dad and I all agreed that surgery was not an option, and we would hope for the best with medical treatment. But, the time had come for us to adhere to the wishes of my mother, to support her decision not to be placed on life support, if it came to that. My mom lay on the gurney agreeing with everything that was said between the doctor and myself. At one point during the conversation, I peered across the gurney, just beyond the doctor, and saw my dad hanging his head in his hands, with tears streaming down his cheeks. We, as a group, were adhering to the end-of-life decisions that had often been discussed, but no one had ever wanted to experience. As I watched my own father grieve, and as I spoke to the physician, I felt the personal anguish that each of my patient's family members experience when I am the one having the conversations with them.

I think that I am a little more sympathetic to these types of situations because of my own personal experiences with my parents. I know how hard it is to make the decision that no one wants to make. I know how hard it is to follow through with family members wishes despite the fact that it will mean that we must give up or let go.

* * *

Ivan had been diagnosed with liver cancer ten weeks before he came to our ICU. His original plan was to go through several sessions of chemotherapy and see what happened, but unfortunately he had only completed a few.

One sunny spring day, Ivan was on his way home from work and found that he could not, physically, make it all the way. He stopped at our emergency room to be seen by a doctor. Ivan was quickly convinced that he was too ill to continue his drive home and was admitted to our ICU. He was suffering from the effects of what we thought, at the time, was sepsis. Sepsis is an infection that has entered the blood stream. We worked to determine the cause of the sepsis. His blood pressure dropped, so vasopressors, Dopamine and Levophed were used to support his blood pressure.

Despite our efforts, within twenty-four hours Ivan deteriorated and required intubation. Ivan spent the next week on maximum support. The ventilator supported his breathing, multiple medications supported his blood pressure, and of course, he had the support of his family. One week later, Ivan was still in the ICU. Despite our efforts, Ivan was now showing signs of kidney failure. Like the lungs, a machine can support the kidneys. Dialysis was the next logical step, but dialysis requires a stable blood pressure and Ivan was not able to achieve that, despite the continuing infusions of medications. Alternative dialysis was the only option. We would start continuous renal replacement therapy (CRRT), a form of dialysis that is done at the bedside twenty-four hours a day. Unlike regular dialysis that is performed for two to four hours each day, CRRT is an around-the-clock treatment that can be done on unstable patients. Now we were supporting his blood pressure, supporting his lungs, and supporting his kidneys.

Within the next few days, his blood pressure started responding to the medications and we were able to slowly wean the vasopressor support. Unfortunately, we had not been as successful at helping his respiratory and his kidney deterioration.

Exactly one week after Ivan came to the ICU, it was my turn to care for him. As I entered the room I first noted that his previously alert and happy personality had vanished. He no longer smiled when his wife kissed him, and he no longer frowned when told that he was going to be suctioned.

Now he simply lay in bed, no longer responding to my voice, no longer accommodating my request to squeeze my hands, and no longer grimacing when I induced painful therapy. The Ivan whom we admitted seven days ago was not in this bed. His skin was becoming golden and the whites of his eyes were yellowing with jaundice caused by his new liver failure. His eyelids lay half open, lacking enough strength to close completely. His body never moved from the strategically placed position that would hopefully prevent pressure sores.

As I was completing my morning assessment, his family arrived, just as they had every morning since his admission. His wife of forty years, his son, and two daughters came religiously as soon as visitors were allowed after shift change. After seeing him, the daily questions started. "Why are his eyes yellow today?"

I explained the jaundice was a result of the toxins that were building up in his liver. The liver was no longer filtering them out of the body. When the liver cannot filter the toxins, we see a change in skin color and the whites of the eyes turn yellow."

"Why are his eyes half-open?"

"He's just very weak, I have put some moisturizing drops in them and I can close them with tape if you want." I tried to offer whatever I could that would make them feel better.

Then the dreaded question, "How's he doing today?"

Many thoughts went through my mind, *what could I give them that would make them happy?* I wanted so bad to tell them he is getting better, but I couldn't. "His blood pressure is stable, it has been stable all night." That's all I had for them that was good. Unfortunately, I had to follow with the bad news that his oxygen level was lower today and we had to increase the oxygen level that we were providing him through the ventilator. I made sure they knew that he wasn't responding to me like he was last time I cared for him.

I couldn't get him to open his eyes, move his fingers or toes, or provide me with any indication that he was willing or able to accommodate my demands. All I got was an occasional blink. As I looked into their eyes, I could see that they were used to hearing bad news. They had quickly become accustomed to hearing disappointing reports.

Despite my reports of his deteriorating consciousness, his wife moved toward the bed and started talking to him. The children stood back and gave mom her space. Eyes drooping with sadness, they watch as their mother shared her love with their dad.

Just outside the room, as I was completing some of the required paperwork, the two eldest children approached. The son turned his sorrowful face toward me, released a sigh and asked the question I'm sure he didn't want to come out of his mouth.

"What do we do now?"

What do you do now? I hate those discussions. They never seem to have a positive outcome—they always seem to end in death. When it gets to the point the family is asking, they already know the answer; they just want someone else to say it. When family members ask this, it's a sure sign that they are starting to realize that this illness is not going to end in the way they were hoping for when the patient first came to the hospital.

"He's not doing well." I tried to open this conversation and see where I should take it.

A nod of both heads confirms that they already knew that.

"His lungs are not working well, but he can live on a ventilator. His kidneys are not functioning, but he can survive with dialysis. But there is no machine that can substitute for the liver. When the liver fails, no machine can take its place."

Another silent nod encouraged me to go on with what I knew had to be brought out in the open.

"Has your dad ever said what he would want in this situation?" This is a question I often ask to initiate a conversation about end-of-life.

Both agreed in harmony that dad would not want machines to keep him alive.

So I initiated what I thought might be the first of the upcoming discussions in response to their "what now" inquiries.

"I don't want you to think I am suggesting anything at this time, but you might want to start thinking about how long you want to continue all of this. Think about what your dad would want."

"What if we don't do all this?" The words from the bravest; the son was taking the role of the decision maker. Later I would find out that this was torturous for him, but he felt he had to be strong for his mother and younger sisters.

"There are options." I progressed slowly, watching their faces, making sure I wasn't going where I shouldn't be.

"You don't have to continue with all this stuff, all these machines. The least we can do is make him a DNR. That means that we continue to do everything we can to make him better, but if his heart stops, we do not do CPR or give him medications to restart the heart."

No words were spoken, but I could see in his facial expressions; he wanted more information, more options, and more choices.

"At some point you might want to start thinking about stopping some of the things we are doing, stopping the dialysis, stopping the medications, and even at some point, maybe even stopping the ventilator."

I could see all of my words were being processed, one by one. I continued as gingerly as I could. At this time, I only wanted to give them enough information to start pondering over, and to start thinking about.

I wanted them to reflect on what dad might want, to let them know that they did have choices, and we could do what dad would want. "You have choices, what is done and what is not."

I could see that both of them were absorbing the new information they had just received. This was a good time to pull back, put it in their hands and let them think and talk alone.

To an ICU nurse, this is a frequent occurrence, but to the average person, this is devastating information and needs to be assimilated and processed and pondered. It is hard for any person to make the decision that may result in ending the life of another, especially if the other is a dearly beloved family member.

Later in the afternoon, the oncologist came to see Ivan. He noted the changes in his consciousness and the increasing jaundice and concluded that Ivan was not going to survive this illness. He told me, before he went to the waiting room to talk to the family, that he was going to tell them that Ivan was not going to survive, and he was going to suggest that we withdraw care. He was going to present the facts to the family and suggest they stop Ivan's suffering.

I shared with the oncologist that I had just had a conversation that morning with two of the children when they presented me with some appropriate questions. They seemed to be starting to think about alternatives to what we were currently doing. I felt they were ready to hear all of their options.

The oncologist told me that he was going to present it as "It's bad for you, but good for your dad." In other words, it's hard for the family to have Ivan die so quickly, but it's better for him to die quickly and not suffer. He spent some time talking to the family, documented his conversation in the notes, and then was off to care for patients in his office.

Shortly after their conversation with the doctor, the family was once again at my side. Mom approached Dad's bedside and begins sobbing as she laid her head on his chest. Sad droopy eyes from the three kids answered my question before I asked it.

"Did the oncologist talk to you?" I knew the answer, but I used that question to open the conversation.

Again, all I received was a quiet nod from the eldest that demonstrated he had been given the bad news.

"Did he tell you it doesn't look good? I inquired, trying to elicit some more information.

Another silent nod, along with tears, was followed by the first of many more specific questions.

"So now what?" Now he wanted specifics, now he wanted me to tell him what he should do. But I couldn't make the decision of what to do. I could give him all the information, I could give him my opinion, but I couldn't take the burden off his shoulders and make the decisions he didn't want to make.

"You have choices." I paused before reminding him of our earlier conversation. "We discussed the option of making him a DNR. If his heart stops, we don't have to do anything—we can let him pass peacefully."

Quickly, he responded positively, "Yes, we want that." That was going to be the easy decision. None of them wanted dad to suffer more than he had to, and none of them wanted dad to be brought back to life if he should die.

I moved forward with more explanations, more options. "Another option is to stop doing everything we're doing to keep him alive." Another pause … to allow for absorption of the options. I continued, "We could stop the dialysis, take the breathing tube out of his lungs and do nothing."

That comment stimulated a need to know exactly what would happen if we did take everything away. He asked how long his dad would live without the breathing tube. That was one answer I didn't have. I tried to explain that I thought initially, he would probably start breathing faster, and then as he tired, he would breath slower and slower until he stopped breathing. If he did start having difficulty breathing, we could give him medications to keep him from struggling. Medications that would relax the muscles, reduces the work of breathing and would keep him comfortable. And, without the supplemental oxygen, the oxygen level in his blood would decrease and the heart, without oxygen, would slow down and eventually stop.

The grimace on his face told me he wasn't sure about that choice. He didn't want to see his dad suffer, even if it would be only for a few minutes. That didn't seem to be the right choice for now, so I continued.

"Another option would be to keep the ventilator on, but stop everything else. We could stop the dialysis and as the toxins build up in the body, the electrolytes will become out of balance and an electrolyte imbalance can also cause the heart to stop." I barely got that sentence out of my mouth and he was once again asking, "How long will that take?"

Again, I was without the exact answer. "It's hard to say, it depends on how quickly the electrolytes and the toxins build up in his body."

He didn't like that answer, but he seemed to like the option of stopping the dialysis better than the previous choice of removing him from the ventilator.

All four family members were gathering around at this time. All were holding on to each other. All were supporting each other both physically and emotionally.

"Let's do that" Once again the eldest took the lead and spoke for the entire family.

"Lets stop dialysis," he reiterated his decision. "What else?" he asked. He needed more choices.

I tried to give them all the choices, as slowly and compassionately as I could. "We can stop the dialysis; we can stop all the medications that are supporting his blood pressure; we can stop drawing lab work if we're not going to treat them anyway; and we can make him a DNR. This will allow him to go peacefully. We don't need to keep doing these procedures if it's not going to help."

"But," I continued, "We will continue to keep him comfortable with pain medications." I wanted to assure them that we would not stop caring for Ivan. We could stop treating him, but would not stop caring for him.

I could see by the facial expressions, this was the best choice. None of them wanted to take a chance that they would have to watch him gasp for breaths when the ventilator was taken away. They continued to hold tightly onto one another as they were making the hardest decision of their life. They were making a decision that would send their dad away. They were, as a group, making the decision that would allow Ivan to leave them peacefully and painlessly.

I needed to confirm what they wanted me to do, and they needed to hear the entire plan once again. So I repeated that we would stop the dialysis, medications, and all lab tests, and if his heart stops, we will not do anything to prolong his suffering and we would allow their dad to go peacefully.

Tears were streaming down all the cheeks now as I explained one more step that I needed to take. Now that we had confirmed what Ivan would want, and decided what the family would support, I needed to call the doctor and tell him about our conversations. I needed to call the doctor so he could give me the orders to do what the family wanted done—nothing.

I left the family, now huddled outside the door, while I phoned the doctor. This time I needed to call Ivan's primary physician, not the oncologist who had initiated this, but the primary physician who hadn't even made rounds yet. I explained to the doctor all the activities of the day, including the conversation the oncologist had with the family. He accommodated me with all the orders I needed; all the orders I needed to stop prolonging Ivan's suffering.

My next call was to the nephrologists, the kidney doctor. I updated him and explained that the family didn't want any more dialysis and he agreed this was the best choice, given the gravity of the situation. I also called the pulmonologist, the lung doctor, to tell him of the DNR order and update him on the status of the situation. Everyone was updated and everyone was agreeable. Now, it was left to me to perform the hardest duties of all.

I stopped the medications and the continuous dialysis. I removed the machines to make room for two chairs at the side of the bed. Two chairs, not four, because that was all that would fit in the small area around the bed. Generally only two family members stay at one time anyway; usually they come and go, staying for a few minutes, then leave so the nurse has room to work.

Ivan's wife didn't want to sit. She remained standing at the side of the bed, bending over him, resting her head on his chest and talking quietly to him. She kept repositioning her arms, under his arm, on his chest, over his head; she couldn't seem to find a spot that was comfortable. She looked across the bed, her sad eyes desperate for help, and said in a pitiful voice. "I just want to hold him, I just want to hold him one more time."

As I saw her anguish, my heart sank, so I immediately started moving things to make that happen. I moved the EKG cable away from his shoulder, I repositioned the oxygen saturation monitor cable from under his arm, and I lifted the ventilator tubing away from his chest to allow her to get closer. I helped her slide her right arm under his weakened upper body and hold onto his shoulder as she reached across his chest with her left arm to hold him close to her chest. Her head snuggled into his neck and she whispered into his ear. I left the room, fighting back tears.

The rest of my shift was spent supporting the family. Ivan was stable for now, providing him with comfort care was my primary goal, and having the family at his side was the best comfort for all of them. The youngest daughter brought in pictures of Ivan; pictures of the entire family at a barbeque in the back yard, pictures of Ivan with his grandchildren. She said she just wanted us to see her dad when he was healthy, to see what he was really like.

In the pictures, I saw a healthy, happy gentleman, smiling and enjoying life with his family. In the bed, I saw a thin, pale yellow, withering, dying old man. It's easier to withdraw care from a pale, dying old man than it is to withdraw care from a healthy looking gentleman. I shared a few memories with his daughter, then smiling, I told her that this was difficult for me and she was making my job harder, because it's harder for me when I see healthy, happy people rather than sick, weak patients.

She seemed to understand my point of view and went on to ask, "Do you guys get desensitized to this?" I'm sure she meant to say, "After so many years in nursing, is death easy for you?" I tried to explain that when I have old patients who have lived a long life, it is usually easier. I can usually rationalize that the older the patient, the better it is for them to die. But, when I have young ones, or those who haven't been ill for a prolonged time, it is still just as hard today as it was twenty years ago. That's when I shared my tears with the family.

I had been supporting them all day while providing Ivan with the comfort measures he needed, but now my shift was over and I was grieving along with them as they prepared to lose their wonderful father.

The next day, after spending the entire night with their father, the family decided it was time to take the next step. They had said their goodbyes and no longer wanted their father to survive on life support machines.

The electrolyte imbalance they had hoped would take his life gently was not happening as rapidly as they wanted. He continued to lie still in the bed, waiting patiently for death. When the doctor came to make rounds in the morning, once again the son was ready to make the next decision.

They wanted the ventilator disconnected and the breathing tube removed from Ivan's throat. They knew that we were all unsure about how he would react to the loss of the breathing support, but it was time to stop the suffering and allow Ivan to be free. The doctor assisted with the removal of the tube. We conferred about what we would do to help Ivan through the last moments of his life. I administered medications in order to assure Ivan would be comfortable during his last breaths.

The tube was removed, Ivan continued to breath without assistance, never providing any signs that he knew any one was watching over him, never giving his family any signal that he was suffering, for another twenty-eight minutes. His wife, his son, and two daughters were holding Ivan and each other. All were sharing their grief, tears of sadness for losing their father and tears of relief for the fact that he was no longer suffering.

This time I could not stay in the room with the family. I had not become desensitized enough to keep my composure while Ivan took his last breaths. I had another six hours to work and I was not able to remain in the room for this painful experience. I gave them space and time to be alone while I kept my distance for my own self-preservation.

Gradually his breathing became slower and slower and his breaths became more and more shallow. As his oxygenation deteriorated, so did his heart rate. As the family sat near his side, Ivan left them.

* * *

To the families—Death is an event we will all have to deal with eventually. Modern technology allows for the healthcare providers to sustain life in many ways, but we must all think about if we would want those machines to keep us alive. Each of us needs to make the decision for ourself, and discuss it with our family. And each of us needs to have the discussion with our parents, our spouse, our children, and anyone about whom we care. We need to know what they want, when the time comes. This needs to be a discussion that we have over and over and over because the more we talk about what each of us wants, the easier it will be to make the decision when the time comes. We must all make our wishes known, so our family will feel better about making that dreaded decision when the time comes.

The ICU nurse deals with death more often than many, but that doesn't make it easier for any of us. Just because we see it more frequently, we never get desensitized, as I was once asked. We do rationalize that it is easier to let go of old people who have lived a full life. Death of the young ones is harder to deal with; they still could have made a difference. Allow us to support you, but allow us to maintain our space in order to maintain our composure.

To the nurses—There are many ways to deal with death and the best way is to make the experience as peaceful and loving as possible. For those patients who we are going to allow to die, the family should be permitted to stay with them as much as possible. Sometimes the visiting rules must be broken if it means a wife will be with her husband during his last breath. Allow more than two visitors in the room at a time if they all want to be there. For those patients for whom we choose to intervene—performing CPR, initiating machines, medications and treatments—make sure that both the patient and family actually want all of our interventions. Make sure the patient and the family is aware of all options. Make sure the family is at the bedside, if they wish to be there, to see what the healthcare providers are doing. Most of all, make sure the dying experience is as gentle as we can make it. We must all consider two critical questions: "What if this were my family?" and "What would I want the nurse to do?" Be a patient advocate and make sure your dying patients and their families have the most peaceful end-of-life experience possible.

You Have A Choice

Your father, or mother, or loved one is admitted to the hospital, he is old and has lived a full life. His work career is over, he has raised a successful family, and has enjoyed several years of retirement. His health had deteriorated over the past few years, and now he has a sudden illness that has landed him in the hospital.

As his condition deteriorates, the doctors tell you he must be moved to the intensive care unit. The nursing staff quickly moves him to another unit that has a lot of patients attached to a lot of machines. There are bells and alarms ringing from every corner. The nurses are scurrying around from bed to bed. You are overwhelmed and unsure of what will happen next.

The nurses approach the bed and start connecting your father to all the machines that hang on the wall. They swarm like bees on honey as they pay undivided attention to your elderly father as he lies in the bed. His breathing is labored, his blood pressure is low, and you don't quite understand what is happening. The nurse explains that she is going to put your dad on some medicine to help his blood pressure and a mask that will help him breath better. If the mask doesn't work, she explains that they—the medical team— might have to put a tube in his throat and attach him to a machine to breath for him. All of this happens very fast and you barely have time to think.

But you *need* to stop and think. You need to think about what your dad wants; medicine for blood pressure support, a mask to help him breath, or a tube in his lungs, attached to a machine. What is it that dad wants? Does he want all these life support measures?

Sometimes all of this happens very quickly and the family doesn't have time to think. Take time to think and to ask questions. You have a choice.

Sometimes the medical team acts rapidly and may not totally explain all the treatments before initiating them. If you know what your dad wants, stop them and ask them to explain each intervention. If the intervention is a life support measure, and you don't want this, tell them. You have a choice.

Sometimes end-of-life interventions are initiated when the family is not present, because there is no other directive to tell the medical team not to do these interventions. If you decide this is not what you want, you can request that these measures be discontinued. You have a choice.

Sometimes families don't discuss end-of-life issues and when dad goes to the hospital medications, tubes, and machines are used to save his life. After a period of time, it becomes apparent that he is not going to get better and the support measures are just prolonging his death. That doesn't mean they must be continued. You have a choice.

You can choose not to initiate any life-support medication, tubes, and machines.

You can choose to withdraw the life-support interventions that have been initiated.

You can choose to have a discussion with all of your family members so you know exactly what they want, when the time comes.

You can choose to deny the fact that your dad is going to get sick, avoid the end-of-life discussion, but it's going to happen eventually.

You can hope it never happens, but eventually it will. The more you *talk* about the choices, the easier it will be to *make* those choices. But it is never easy, even when it's not your own family.

CHAPTER 13

Resurrection—
When They Come Back

*When the patients get better and leave the ICU, we
often don't know where they go.*

Resurrection, the act of bringing the dead back to life. Some
people believe in resurrection, some believe in a life after death, and
some believe in some form of living beyond death. Because the ICU
is where the sickest patients struggle to survive, it would be expected
that the frequency of death is higher than any other area of the
hospital. But not everyone who comes to ICU dies. The ICU patients come from surgery, from the emergency room, or from the
other floors of the hospital. They come to our unit because they
need a different level of care, and interventions that cannot be accomplished on other units. Some patients are on ventilators to help
them breath, some need specialized monitoring or supportive medications, and some simply need a higher level of observation. These
patients, once stabilized, progress to the point where they can be
transferred to the medical or surgical units. They continue their
recovery and go home.

We, the ICU nurses, often don't know what happens to most of
our patients after they leave us. Occasionally, different nurses will

befriend specific patients, usually those who were unfortunate enough to spend a longer than normal time in the ICU. After the patient is transferred out to the medical floor, some nurses will visit the patient upstairs and report back to her co-workers. We like to know how they are healing and that our hard work was a success. We also enjoy the news that our previously dangerously ill patient is being discharged. Some patients are in our unit for a long time. They are critically ill, stabilized, and transferred, but we never know what happens to them after they roll out of our unit.

* * *

Bennett was a healthy looking fifty-two-year-old male. He arrived in the emergency room with complaints of shortness of breath and fever. He had been suffering from a normal winter cold and had been feeling worse the past few days. While in the emergency room, Bennett developed severe respiratory distress related to what we quickly learned was pneumonia. He was intubated and admitted to the ICU. The tube placed in his throat, connected to a ventilator, would help Bennett breathe until his pneumonia cleared.

This is not an uncommon occurrence. Patients with severe cases of pneumonia may become hypoxic (suffer from a lack of oxygen) and require ventilator support. As the pneumonia improves, the ventilator support is weaned off and the patient is on his way to recovery. Usually this happens with elderly patients, not healthy fifty-two-year-old men. Unfortunately for Bennett, his pneumonia was so severe that he could not be treated with a course of antibiotics. His condition had deteriorated to the point where he needed ventilator support in order to survive this sudden illness.

Initially, we thought that we could wean Bennett off the ventilator in a few days. Once the antibiotics did their job, he would get better. The ventilator would no longer be needed, and he would be transferred upstairs to the medical floor to continue his antibiotic therapy. In a week or so, he would go home. Unfortunately, the plan of care did not progress as we wanted it to. Soon after initiating ventilator support, Bennett's mental status changed. Bennett had a history of bipolar disease, also known as Manic-Depressive disorder. People with bipolar disease experience periods of mental mania, hyperactive states, followed by periods of depression. The mental status of these patients is managed delicately with medications. Now that Bennett was in the ICU, unable to take his usual medications, it didn't take long for his bipolar disease to affect his mentation.

Over a period of days, the awake and alert Bennett gradually turned into a stuporous, somber creature. He slowly became unresponsive to any of our attempts to stimulate him. He no longer communicated with his nurses or his wife. He would simply lie in bed; receive the breaths we provided him, and make no attempt to interact. He would gaze into the air, move when stimulated, but not seemingly responding to anything the nurses or his wife asked of him. After about a week, we were puzzled. This was not right. Bennett came in, walking and talking, and now he was indifferent. Despite the fact that we had resumed all of the medications he had been taking at home, Bennett was not responding, as we wanted him to. He was not the same Bennett who walked into the emergency room a short week ago. Despite the fact that his pneumonia seemed to be clearing, we could not wean him from the ventilator.

We work hard, the doctors and nurses, to regain normal health for our patients. Our goal is to return all patients to their normal state of health. Sometimes, though, despite all our efforts, we can't achieve our goal.

What was going on with Bennett? Perhaps it was just one of those flukes when things just don't go right. Maybe it was one of those cases where the doctor tells you that ninety-nine percent of the time everything goes well, but that one percent of the time, the unexpected may happen. The reason for Bennett's delayed recovery was not apparent, but we had him in our unit and we would continue to care for him until we could figure it out and help him return home to his wife and his active life.

Several weeks into Bennett's stay, it became apparent that we were not going to be able to wean him from the ventilator. We cared for him until we established that he was going to be dependent on that ventilator for an extended amount of time, possibly for the rest of his life. After repeated weaning attempts were unsuccessful, we started preparing for long-term ventilator care. Bennett needed to be transferred out of our acute care facility to a long-term ventilator facility, a facility where they specialize in caring for patients who are ventilator dependent. A place where he could live for a long time, attached to the machine that would keep him alive.

In order to prepare him for his new home, we performed a tracheostomy, placed the breathing tube directly through his neck, so the ET tube could be removed from his mouth. We inserted a feeding tube directly into his stomach, to maintain his nutritional needs now that he was no longer able to eat a normal meal. After several more weeks in our ICU, Bennett was transferred to a local long-term care facility. Maybe he was going to spend the rest of his life attached to that machine. Maybe he was never going to communicate the way he used to. Maybe we would never know.

✳ ✳ ✳

Our job, in the acute care ICU, is to care for the patients, get them better and discharge them to another floor for continued care and discharge planning. Occasionally, we have patients who do not recover, as we want them to. Some patients do not get well enough to move to the medical floor in anticipation of discharge. Some of our patients require extended lengths of stay and will continue to require long-term care. These patients are discharged to extended care facilities for long-term care. We care for them throughout their critical hours; we stabilize them but cannot manage to find the right way to wean them from the ventilator. We send them off to another facility and never see them again. Some of the local facilities will send letters, updating us on the progress of the patients we transfer to them, but some facilities don't. Sometimes, in passing conversation, one nurse might say to another "I wonder what ever happened to ..." Too often, all we can do is wonder.

✳ ✳ ✳

One fall day, six or seven months after Bennett left us, I was at the bedside of my patient and one of my co-workers came to get me. She pulled me away telling me that I needed to come to the hallway to see who was there. I walked around the corner to see a tall, healthy looking, now fifty-three-year-old man. I looked at him and saw a happy face. His grin went from ear to ear. He was greeting everyone who gathered around him. I looked again, but didn't recognize the person who was standing in our hallway. Just as I heard someone say his name, a name that I remember hearing almost daily several months ago, I glanced to his side and immediately recognized his wife. I recognized the woman who had so diligently spent every day at his side. I did not, however, recognize this healthy looking man. But of course, he was now walking and talking and looking great. His color was good, his hair was clean, and his muscles were strong. I remembered seeing a sick, pale, non-communicative soul attached to machines. I had never seen him in this condition. This was not the same person I remembered as Bennett.

Happiness filled that hallway. It was so great to see one of our successes. Every nurse had questions. "Tell us what happened" "Where did you go?" "How long did you stay?" "How are you now?" Too many questions, Bennett couldn't answer, but his wife could.

She filled us in. After his two-month stay with us, he went to the long-term care facility. He stayed there another two months, and was eventually weaned off the ventilator and was able to start some aggressive rehabilitation. Because of his extended time in bed, he had to regain strength in his muscles, sitting, walking and building strength. He ate meals and drank supplements to regain the thirty pounds that he had lost during the four months of his hospitalization. Eventually she was able to take her husband back home with her. Another few weeks and he was back to his old self. It had been established that Bennett's bipolar disease had indeed been the cause of his change in mentation. A combination of the pneumonia and the bipolar disease had caused an unexpectedly long recuperation time.

Bennett did not remember any of his ICU stay. He didn't remember coming to the hospital, he didn't remember being in our unit, and he didn't remember any of the smiling faces that were now gawking at him on this day. We assured him that it was probably a good thing that he didn't remember our dungeon-like ICU or us. It was OK that he didn't remember us, we remembered him.

His wife brought him into our ICU that day. She wanted to show him off. She wanted to show the nurses what he was really like. "This is my husband," she said with a broad smile. "This is the real Bennett, not the starry-eyed slug all of you saw in your ICU bed." We all gathered around Bennett as if he was a trophy. His wife was proud, but so were we. We were proud to see that our hard work had paid off. The negative affects often occur right before our eyes, but we don't always get to see the positive ones. We need to see the positive endings in order to balance the negative. Now we could see with our own eyes, what we try so hard, everyday, to accomplish. Bennett had been resurrected. Once, we almost gave up on him, but he came back to us alive and well.

* * *

Paul, a 49-year-old physician, was visiting from out of town when he developed severe nausea and vomiting. Paul was suffering from pancreatitis, an inflammation of the pancreas. After being tormented with a multitude of tests, he was informed that his liver was failing. It didn't take long for Paul to deteriorate. His pancreas was not working, his liver was failing, and within twenty-four hours, his breathing efforts also became compromised. Paul was placed on life support, a ventilator to help him breath. He became septic, developed an infection throughout his blood stream, resulting in dangerously low blood pressure; his body was in shock. Only a few days after walking into our hospital, Paul was clinging to life with a multitude of machines and medications keeping him alive.

We continued to do everything we could to help Paul regain his normal life. We did what we could just to keep him alive. Despite all our efforts, he was not improving. Several weeks into his treatment, after establishing that we had exhausted all of our available resources, we started looking for other options. We searched the area for another local facility that could provide additional options for this young dying man. After working non-stop, day and night, with no improvement, we transferred the sick doctor to a local teaching hospital, which could hopefully save his life.

In order to facilitate rapid transport, we arranged for helicopter transportation, accompanied by a team of expert nurses and physicians. Ambulance by highway would take too long and would not be safe. We assisted the receiving team as they prepared him for transport. We provided all the test results and reports that we had completed. We did what we could and now we were handing him to another group of specialists in hopes that they could restore his health.

As Paul was being removed from our unit, we pleaded with his family to keep us informed of his condition. His wife assured us she would call. But days and weeks went by and no one heard from her. After a while, we could only assume that the outcome was not good. Who would expect a wife to call the ICU and tell us that her husband had died? He was so critically ill, so unstable, that most likely the reason we didn't hear from his family was because they couldn't bear to give us the bad news, the news we didn't want to hear.

Five weeks after we sent Paul off in that helicopter, many of us had resolved ourselves to the fact that he had probably passed. But suddenly, one sunny afternoon, he walked back into our unit. This time he walked in smiling and happy. Unlike the original entrance, on a gurney suffering from intractable vomiting, this time he looked healthy and happy. His wife was by his side, smiling almost as generously as her husband. Paul had gone to the teaching hospital where they provided him with a treatment option that was not available in our facility and after a few weeks, he was back on his feet and ready to go back to work.

All of the nurses gathered around to see how wonderful "our" patient looked. This gentleman, who we all assumed had died, was now standing in our unit, conversing with the nurses who had worked hard to save his life. He was walking and talking and most of all laughing and feeling good. Once again, we were excited to see one of our patients resurrected. One who we had almost given up on, one who we had decided was no longer alive, was indeed alive and well.

* * *

Bennett and Paul were both in our ICU suffering from life-threatening illnesses. Both were provided all the care we could provide, but despite our care, they did not do what we wanted them to do. They did not get better. Both were eventually transferred to another facility. We lost contact with each of them and could only assume that those two sick patients had succumbed to the devastating illnesses we tried hard to cure. But, eventually, both of these patients came back to show the nurses in the ICU they were alive and well, and happy to grace us with their healthy presence. Bennett and Paul, who we thought had died, were alive and well. Both had come back to give us the rewards we strive to achieve. Both, in our eyes, had been resurrected.

CHAPTER 14

Peace and Tranquility

Having a family member in the ICU is stressful. How
the nurse can help alleviate the stress.

When a patient comes into the ICU, it's a stressful event for everyone involved. The patient is stressed, if they are awake enough to know where they are. The family is stressed because they have just been told that their loved one is sick enough to require intensive care, And, the nurse is stressed because she has just received, yet another unstable patient. Stress can cause many emotions; different people react to stress in different ways. Some cry, some laugh, some withdraw, and others act out with a variety of behaviors.

When family members enter the unit, they are entering a frightful place. They enter the room with eyes wide open; seeing things that may not be meant for the average eyes, hearing sounds that are disturbing to most, and feeling emotions that are uncomfortable for the majority. Most of these family members have never experienced a place like this. We, the ICU nurses, are comfortable with all of the sounds and sights because we have grown accustomed to each of them. We know exactly when we can turn away from the tones that are simply meant to alert the nursing staff, and when to call for help because the tone is indicative of a life-threatening emergency. We know which alarms need our attention, which bell is more important than others, and which tone can be ignored and stored in our memory banks. We are familiar with all the sounds; moans and groans of semi-conscious patients, sobs from grieving family members, incoherent attempts at conversations from the confused elderly, and irrelevant conversations between two staff members.

The family members, on the other hand, hear all of this chaos, the multiple conversations and each of the many alarms and buzzers. They react whether they realize it or not, to every one of these unfamiliar sounds. They don't know any better so they assume that each of the alarms are life-threatening, each of the sounds are catastrophic, and each of the conversations must be about their own family member.

The goal of the nurse is to decipher all the sounds and noises while providing care for the patients. She must also support the family during this traumatic time. In order to provide a tranquil setting for patients and family, we remain calm and address every situation in a caring, competent, and communicative manner.

* * *

Camille was a sixty-eight-year-old woman who was in the ICU for chronic obstructive pulmonary disease (COPD). She was on a ventilator because without it, she could not breath. Her daughter, Brenda, would come to visit every day. She was obviously concerned that her mother was not getting better as fast as she expected, and she wanted to make sure that all of her mom's needs were being met. Rather than building a rapport with the nurses, and having daily discussions about her mom's progress, and what could be done to help, Brenda always seemed to voice her concerns in a negative manner. Every day when she came to visit, it seemed that she would look for things to complain about. All the nurses could expect a list of complaints. "Her gown has a spot on it." "Her hair hasn't been combed before breakfast." "She needs more lotion on her feet." "She needs to be off this machine."

Unfortunately, the staff quickly built up a shield and they would try to avoid her so they wouldn't have to listen to what they felt were unreasonable demands from an unreasonable family pest. She would make demands that were not always possible to meet, and would not back down when the nurses tried to provide explanations for many of her concerns. When informed of the plan of care, Brenda would criticize the staff and claim that everyone was incompetent. It seemed that no matter what we did, or how hard we tried, we were not going to make her happy.

One day, when the doctor was making rounds, Brenda requested that her mother get a television. She felt that her mother needed a television to help her relax and she was sure a television would help her breathe better. The doctor suggested, to the nurse, that we try to move Camille into one of our private rooms that had a television. Unfortunately, the doctor suggested that option in the presence of Brenda and she assumed that it would be done. Many think, if the doctor says it, it will be done—as simple as that.

The next day, when Brenda came to visit, she immediately became angry and started complaining that her mother was not yet in a private room and still did not have a television. The nurse tried to respond to her initially by saying that we don't have televisions in the ICU. She was unable to continue her explanation when Brenda quickly snapped back with "Well, you just don't care," and turned and walked away. Camille's nurse was bothered by the event, came to me and told me that the daughter didn't even give her a chance to finish what she was trying to say before she just stormed out of the unit.

Within minutes, I received a call from the hospital operator telling me that she had a family member on the phone who wanted to speak to someone in charge. I found out quickly that it was Brenda and started dreading the fact that I was the charge nurse on the day this daughter had decided to cause a larger than usual fuss. She started, very abruptly, by informing me that the doctor had promised her mother a television the previous day and she was demanding to know why it had not been done. Then she went on to insist that if her mother was not going to get a television in the current unit, she should be moved to the other ICU that had televisions. Her tone of voice was very demeaning; she spoke very quickly, not allowing me to answer any questions before she barked more. After I listened to each and every one of her complaints and questions, I calmly started to explain the situation to her. I reiterated that we only had two rooms with televisions and patients who required private rooms for isolation purposes currently occupied each of those. We did have another unit that the doctor had suggested we move her mother to, but that unit did not have the high level of visibility the current unit had. I explained to her that her mother was sick enough that she required a higher level of observation and to move her to the other unit would not be in the best interest for her recovery; the other unit was not a good option. I continued to explain that one of the private rooms with a television may soon be empty and if I could accommodate moving her mother into that room, I would. But I also informed her that if we had a patient who was admitted, and needed the private room because of isolation, that I would have to move her mother out of that private room at that time. In the meantime, I would assure that our portable stand, with a VCR player could be rolled over to her mother's bedside, and she could watch movies. I enlisted her help to obtain some movies that her mom would enjoy, and assured her that we would accommodate her wishes and assist with the movies as needed.

After I took the time to explain the situation to Brenda, the reasons why her mother had not been moved to the private room, and the alternatives, she calmed down. I enlisted her help in making sure her mother got what she felt she needed. We also spent some time discussing her mother's condition and her care. I tried to explain all of the treatments we were doing and the progress we were making. I reassured Brenda that we were doing the best we could for her mother. When she expressed concerns that her mother was not recuperating as fast as she had in the past, I reminded her that as a person ages, the body regenerates more slowly. Therefore, it takes longer to recuperate.

After I spent time explaining and consoling Brenda, she was no longer angry and was more cooperative with the nurses caring for her mom. Brenda was an example of how many family members react when they think their mother or father is not getting what they think is best for them. Not knowing the entire situation, not having all the information, and not being able to control the surroundings causes stress and many react in negative ways.

* * *

Stress and anxiety create many unwanted emotions. When a person feels like they are out of control, they may act out. In the healthcare environment, if a patient or family member feels wronged by the healthcare team, they speak out; they complain to anyone and everyone who will listen, in an attempt to make their wrong a right. How each of us avoids, or regains control of uncontrollable situations depends on how we present ourselves during the initial situation or when trying to resolve the situation.

I believe that if the nurses are caring, competent and communicative they can prevent these unwanted outbursts, which cause even more stress for all involved. Caring shows that the nurse really is concerned about the patient and the needs of the family. Being attentive to the needs, even the most minor ones, is important. Nurses care, by nature, that's why they are in this profession. But some nurses have a more caring, compassionate personality and show that they care more than others. If the nurse is short or abrupt with the patient or the family, they will interpret that as not caring. Any patient, who is lying in bed, totally dependent on the nurse, wants someone who cares about them. Nurses who demonstrate this caring manner will have an advantage over those who are unable to show how much they care.

Competence demonstrates that the nurse knows what she is doing. Showing the patient and the family members that she is confident in her skills and in what she knows is reassuring. If she presents herself in a manner that appears that she doesn't know what she's doing, the patient and the family will lose confidence in the care that is being provided. If the nurse is unsure of any task that she is required to do, she should ask for assistance and clarification before going to the bedside. No one wants a nurse caring for them who doesn't seem to know what she is doing.

Communication promotes understanding of all events for the patient and the family. The nurse must constantly explain what she is doing and why she is doing each task. She must answer all of the questions when they are asked. If the family members ask a question and the nurse is reluctant to answer, doubt will be instilled in their minds. If, however, she is forthcoming with information, shares what she knows, and shares her opinion, the patient and the family will have more confidence in her and the care they are receiving.

* * *

Rita was a sixty-year-old woman who was admitted to the ICU with asthma. Within a few hours of admission, Rita's condition had deteriorated. She was working harder and harder to breath and was rapidly deteriorating toward a respiratory arrest. Her doctor decided the only thing to do for Rita was to intubate her, insert a breathing tube into her lungs. Without intubation, she would surely have died.

When intubating any patient, the doctor inserts a scope into the patient's throat, visualizes the trachea and gently pushes the soft breathing tube through the scope into the main airway. After positioning the tube, the doctor withdraws the scope, leaving the tube in the airway. This routine procedure was uneventful for Rita and she was placed on a ventilator. For several hours, it looked as if Rita's course of care would be routine. Ventilator support for a few days, increase in steroids, commonly used for respiratory ailments, and once over the difficult period, we would wean her from the ventilator and she would return home.

Unfortunately, for Rita, this plan was soon modified. Hours after the intubation, Rita developed complications and her condition deteriorated. The physician was at the bedside, interventions were initiated rapidly and tests and x-rays were done. Despite our efforts, Rita was not responding to our treatments. Rita was sedated in order to control her breathing patterns with the mechanical support. Because of the sedation, she could not express her concerns, but her son, Jesse, was there to do that for her. Jesse was experiencing a new kind of stress; he was watching his mother deteriorate before his eyes. What could he do? He could not tell the doctors what to do, because he wasn't trained. He could not tell the nurses what to do, because he didn't know what was normal. He was helpless; he could only ask questions.

"What's happening to my mom? Why is she like this? What have you done? Have you done the right thing? What are you going to do?" Question after question came from Jesse's mouth while the doctor and several nurses were working diligently to save the life of his mother. Because the nurse at the bedside was not answering Jesse's questions to his satisfaction, his stress level was building and his confidence in his mom's care was falling.

In order to get answers, Jesse decided to ask others, anyone who would tell him what he needed to hear. He first asked to speak to the charge nurse; she didn't give him the answers he wanted. He next demanded to talk to the nursing supervisor. The supervisor tried to explain what was happening to his mother, but he still wasn't happy. Eventually, during his all night struggle, Jesse became angry and upset. By morning, he was barely approachable. He was furious because his mother was critically ill, and seemed sicker now than she was when she came to the hospital, and he was distraught because he had no control over the sequence of events. He was experiencing a normal stressful experience that many go through in the ICU.

When I came on duty, fresh and rested in the morning, an exhausted, frustrated nurse who had worked all night to save Rita's life greeted me. She was relieved to know that her shift was near the end. She was thankful that she would no longer have to deal with Jesse while she struggled to do her job. She thoroughly explained the sequence of events that she had suffered through all night. We reviewed the physical assessment and the plan of care for my new patient. Before she left, she felt she needed to warn me about Rita's son, who had been causing trouble all night. She informed me that he was not happy with her care. She went on to say that he had asked the same questions over and over and would not listen to anything she told him. She reported that he was rude. She suggested that if I knew what was best, I would try to avoid him because he had been complaining all night long to the charge nurse, the nursing supervisor, and anyone who would listen.

When receiving a report like this, I usually listen carefully, but try not to jump to conclusions. Some family members react to stress differently, some nurses do not communicate as well as others, and there are always two sides to every story. I take in all the facts and sort through the opinions and wait to make my own conclusions.

After receiving report, I immediately performed a thorough assessment of the patient. I reviewed the orders, set my priorities and made a tentative plan for the day. Within minutes of assuming my assignment, the son entered the room. As he approached, I noticed a tired, unshaven, puffy-eyed young man. Beneath his warn out physical appearance I sensed a distrusting scowl coming from his face and an aura of anger fuming from his entire being. My first thought was, *Oh boy, here comes trouble.* He already looks like he's ready to tear me apart. How was I going to handle this guy and his mom too? So, I decided to just start from the beginning and see what happened.

I stopped what I was doing, extended my right hand offering to shake and introduced myself. I informed him that I would be there all day with his mother. I clarified the current status of his mother's condition. I told him what I saw, what I heard, and what I thought. I explained all of the medications that were infusing through the IV pumps and what each was doing to make his mom better. I reiterated the function of the machines in the room, the monitor and the ventilator. As he fixated on the bedside monitor, I explained what the waveforms and numbers represented. Then I shared with him my plan of care and my goals for that day.

Maybe it was my imagination, but it appeared that, with a quiet sigh, his entire body relaxed and his face was no longer taught and stiff. I had just given him the tools he needed to reduce his stress level. I had just given him all the information I had. Now he knew what was happening and where we were going. Perhaps being caught up in the unsettling events of the night prevented the other staff from providing Jesse with what he needed—reassurance. Perhaps the nurses and the doctors were so busy doing tasks to prevent death that they didn't have the time to give Jesse the information that would allow him to see more clearly. Maybe the priorities were to care for Rita and worry about Jesse later. Whatever the reason, the needs of this man were not met and because of his exorbitant stress level, he had been acting out all night long. And now he had been labeled a troublemaker.

During the morning hours, we continued with the multiple interventions that would help Rita. Each of her doctors, primary care provider, pulmonologist, and now surgical consultant were in and out of the room many times. More and more tests and discussions filled the busy morning. After the situation was stabilized and the medical plan was established, the physicians sat and talked with Jesse, once again.

Now he was given the medical interpretation of the critical events that had occurred during the night and he was given medical opinions. After fourteen long hours, Jesse now was completely informed and no longer felt alienated by the medical team he had been bucking all night long.

Rita had developed a rare complication that required immediate surgical interventions. This specific high-level surgical procedure was not available at our facility. Rita needed to be transferred to a local University Hospital where they could provide the higher-level of service. Jesse was anxious to make the transfer happen as soon as possible, but not more anxious than we were. We initiated the search for a physician, a hospital and all of the red tape that was necessary to make it happen.

Jesse wanted his mother to go to the best facility for her specific needs, and he wanted this as soon as possible. Unfortunately, this was not possible and the transfer was delayed. What we thought would be a simple transfer, via helicopter and a critical care transport team, did not occur as we expected. We worked diligently all day calling different facilities and trying to expedite a swift relocation for Rita. I worked all day supporting Rita physically and Jesse psychologically. I continued to share every bit of information I had with him. Each time we contacted another facility, I would inform him. Each time we received a denial, I consoled him. Each time there was another disappointing delay, I supported him.

Throughout the day, Jesse and I developed an understanding. I would work hard to provide the best care possible for his mother. I would keep him informed of each change, and I would include him in all of the decisions. I also made sure that my caring, competent, communicative skills were displayed clearly for Jesse. Not only did I make sure he knew I cared about his mother and her condition, I made sure he knew that I cared about him and his concerns. I provided quality care for Rita, I displayed no doubts and I explained everything that I was doing. This demonstrated my competence in my nursing abilities. And, finally, I communicated everything with Jesse. I told him every minute detail, every change and every update, no matter how big or small.

Rita was finally transferred to that University Hospital later that evening. Jesse was at her bedside as the transport team readied her for the forty-mile helicopter ride. I made sure the nurse from the transport team explained the process to Jesse, and made sure he had the directions and the location of where his mother would be, once arriving to the new facility. As Rita was rolling out of the unit, Jesse came to me. He thanked me for taking good care of his mother and for all of my hard work. He told me he appreciated everything I had done for her.

I graciously accepted his gratitude and wished him the best of luck. I asked him to call us in a few days to let us know how his mom was doing. With this, I was reiterating that we truly cared about his mother and her condition. I walked him out of the unit, made sure he had his driving directions and gave him a gentle hug as he left to embark on another stressful situation with his mother.

By the end of the day, I saw a different person than the one I was warned about at the beginning of my shift. I did not see an angry troublemaker. I saw a gentle, compassionate, worried family member who was concerned about the survival of his mother. I saw a relaxed son who was now confident we had done everything possible to protect the survival of someone he loved dearly.

* * *

I feel strongly that if I give my all to my patients and their family members, they will be happy and each case will be a success. Sometimes unfortunate complications occur, but if the patient and the family feel they received the best care, they will accept those bad outcomes more easily.

The ICU is a stressful place, for nurses, for patients, and for families. Nurses must work through their own stress and provide stress relief for the others, especially the family members. If the patients or the family members are not comfortable, either with the care received or the patient's progress, their stress level will increase. If they are worried, they will act out. They will reach out for whatever help or attention they can get.

Commonly this is in the form of complaining to whomever will listen and whoever they feel will resolve the situation. They will complain to charge nurses, they will complain to supervisors and they will complain to administrators.

Complaints are good if they serve a purpose. But, it is our goal to avoid complaints and provide quality care for the patients and informative support to the families. No one deliberately ignores the family, or harms the patient. Healthcare providers strive to heal. Their goal is to cure, but sometimes that is not possible. Lack of knowledge and lack of confidence may precipitate frustration. Providing the patients and the families with the knowledge they need and the support they need is part of our job. Provide them with the caring, competent, communicative support that they deserve during this stressful time. Treat them like they are your family. Treat them the way each of us would want to be treated, to maintain peace and tranquility in the ICU.

Is Competent Enough?

Or do we need to be Caring and Communicative too?

Sally and Sue are both nurses. Each is competent in her nursing ability. Each of them handles the same situation in a different way.

* * *

Sally was taking care of Joe. Joe came to the ICU after experiencing some chest pain. He had never experienced chest pain in the past. He kept saying that he was not feeling pain; it was a squeezing sensation across his shoulders. After a thorough examination in the emergency room, Joe was admitted to the ICU. Joe was assigned a cardiologist who happened to be on call when he arrived. He had never met the man before this hospital stay.

His wife, Jane, was very nervous and scared about this new change in Joe's health. Jane sat at the side of the bed all day and tried to learn what was happening with her husband. Sally entered the room, did not acknowledge Jane and asked Joe if he had any chest pain. He replied "no" so she told him if he needs anything call her.

Later that day, the unfamiliar cardiologist visits. He told Joe there was a test he needed to do to see if he has any blocked coronary arteries. He told Joe he had scheduled the test for later that day. Joe and his wife agreed to have the test and were looking forward to discovering the results to see what exactly was happening.

When the nurse brought the consent form into the room for Joe to sign, she simply said, "Here is the form you must sign to have the test." Joe signed and the nurse went back to the nurses' station to finish her conversation with her friends.

A few hours later, Jane was at the bedside when the team came to take Joe for the procedure. She said to the nurse, "I'm just so scared, I don't know what to expect."

The nurse replied "Don't worry, he'll be fine" and Joe went down the hall for the procedure.

* * *

Sue was taking care of John. John came to the ICU after experiencing some chest pain. He had never experienced chest pain in the past. He kept saying that he was not feeling pain—it was a squeezing sensation across his shoulders. After a thorough examination in the emergency room, John was admitted to the ICU. John was assigned a cardiologist who just happened to be on call in the emergency room on the evening he came. He had never met the man before this hospital stay. His wife, Judy, was very nervous and scared about this new change in John's health. Judy sat at the side of the bed all day and tried to learn what was happening with her husband. Sue entered the room and greeted Judy and John. Sue asked Joe if he had any chest pain. He replied "no" so she explored further. "Any pressure, or tightness, or any abnormal feelings?"

"Well, yes, I still have some squeezing sensation, but it's in my shoulders, not my chest."

Sue explains to John and Judy that typically the discomfort felt when having a heart attack is called chest pain, but often the feeling is more like a tightness, pressure, or squeezing, and the discomfort is not always in the chest, sometimes it is in the neck, jaw and arms. Sue continued to encourage John to let her know if he had any abnormal discomfort, because any discomfort was important and she wanted to treat it. John agreed, and Sue moved on to other tasks.

Later that day, the unfamiliar cardiologist visited. Sue followed him into the room because she knew John and Judy were anxious and she wanted to assure that all of their questions were answered and all of their concerns were addressed. The cardiologists told John there was a test he needed to do to see if he had any blocked coronary arteries. He told John he had scheduled the test for later that day. As the unfamilar cardiologist started to leave the room, Sue asked John and his wife if they had any questions for the doctor. Each of them, now that they had permission to inquire, asked several questions. "How will you do the test?" "When will we get the results?" "What will we need to do if blockages are found?" "When could John expect to go home?" All of their questions were answered before the physician left the room. Now John and Judy knew exactly what to expect and could relax.

When the nurse brought the consent form into the room for John to sign, she stopped and asked if either of them had any more questions. After answering a few more questions and assuring they were comfortable, she had John sign the consent and told him if anything else came to mind, be sure to ask.

A few hours later, Judy is at the bedside when the team came to take John for the procedure. She said to the nurse, "I'm just so scared, I hope everything goes OK."

The nurse replied, "I'm sure you are scared, this is all new to you. The procedure should take about an hour. If you want, you can wait in the waiting room and as soon as the procedure is done, someone will come out and get you. If you have any questions, I'll be here, you can come and ask me." Sue gave Judy a comforting smile as she walked beside the gurney, with John, to the x-ray department.

* * *

There are several types of nurses. Some are like Sally and some are like Sue. Sally provides competent care. Sue provides competent care along with a caring manner and she communicates with her patients.

CHAPTER 15

By Day and By Night

When a nurse is asked
to be a nurse when off duty.

A nurse is a nurse at all times. When I went to school to become a nurse, I didn't realize I would be a nurse twenty-four hours a day. I thought I was going to school to get an education that I could use during normal working hours to help others. I didn't realize that my career choice would be a life choice that would follow me everywhere, at all times.

Many professional skills are applied in routine, day-to-day activities. A chef can cook dinner for the family; an electrician can rewire his own home or that of a friend's; a mechanic can help repair cars for family members.

However, is the chef expected always to barbecue the burgers at the picnics? Is the electrician permanently on call for every neighborhood malfunction? And does the mechanic repair all the cars in the parking lot at the shopping mall? Only a nurse is expected to be a "nurse" at all times. If a family member is ill, the nurse is called. If a car hits a neighbor child, the nurse is summoned. And if a stranger collapses and needs CPR, the nurse is quickly pushed to the front of the crowd. I'm not suggesting this is bad, it just seems to be a natural occurrence.

Perhaps it's the respect that nurses have gained, the honor they carry that promotes the idea that they are the one who should be called upon when help is needed and when a medical opinion is necessary. Or maybe, it's that we, who choose the nursing profession, have the natural instinct to help others when we notice someone is in need. When it comes to a person's health, or life, not everyone can provide the expert, sometimes life and death care, that a nurse can provide. Many health-related concerns are urgent, so people don't want to wait until later to obtain answers or support. Thus, the nurse is summoned immediately, any time of the day or night.

✳ ✳ ✳

One of my son's teammates was playing baseball when he was hit with a pitched fastball. Just before the ball contacted his back, he swung himself around and protected his back with his hand. Thus, the fastball clobbered his wrist. He immediately fell to the ground in pain and was removed from play. For the rest of the game, he iced his injury as instructed by his coaches.

After the game, his parents coaxed him to come to me, the nurse who could tell them what to do. As they were approaching, his dad was saying "I think it's broken, I think we should go to the hospital."

Meanwhile Mom was whining quietly to me, "I don't want to spend my Friday night in the emergency room."

I examined the wrist. It was red, but that was most likely from the ice. There was no swelling, but he seemed to be in significant pain. He wouldn't allow me to flex his wrist because it caused too much discomfort. He could flex his fingers and his thumb but again refused to move the wrist at all. I couldn't be sure there were no broken bones, but I certainly didn't see anything that convinced me that there was.

Dad continued insisting on a trip to the hospital, while Mom was making excuses not to go. After some bantering back and forth, they both looked at me and asked what I thought they should do.

Having three sons of my own, experiencing many sports injuries, and occasionally working a shift in the emergency department, helped me to make my decision.

I explained to them that I could not be sure that there weren't any broken bones, but my gut feeling was that he had a soft tissue injury. The wrist was hit hard, there was a lot of pain, but it was probably just a bruise. I told them that, based on my experience, the emergency room is very busy in the evenings, and I personally, would not want to wait several hours for an x-ray that might show nothing was wrong. If there were any broken bones, the doctor would immobilize it and refer him to an orthopedist. They wouldn't be able to see an orthopedist until Monday. My official nursing opinion was to splint the wrist, ice it off and on throughout the evening, and see how it looked the next morning. If it was still just as sore, or swollen, then go to the emergency room first thing in the morning when there would be less of a wait.

Both parents agreed on the plan. They followed me home after the game so I could loan them one of the many wrist immobilizers that I had in my supply of sports injury equipment. Mom thanked me for saving her from a trip to the hospital, and Dad thanked me for my opinion despite the fact that he still wasn't sure I was right.

The next morning, I phoned and talked to the mom. She assured me that her son's wrist was fine, and informed me that dad and son were on their way to our house to return the immobilizer. Within minutes, I was once again examining the wrist. Fifteen hours after the suspected fracture, the wrist was feeling fine, no pain, no problems flexing, and the son was on his way to play baseball once again.

Friends ask opinions. I can only give opinions based on my education and experience. I often tell them that, officially my opinion is worth what they pay for it, nothing. Unofficially, my opinion is worth what a mother of three boys, with some education and experience can provide. My professional opinion for that injury was correct, that time I was right.

* * *

Unlike the next time, when once again at the baseball fields, my nursing opinion was requested. A high fly ball was hit into the stands. Just as we heard a "crack," everyone gasped. The high fly ball had landed solidly on the top of a mother's head. My instincts made me walk to the other side of the field to make sure the victim of the ill-placed baseball was all right. As I was standing back, watching from afar, I was suddenly pushed to the front of the crowd. "She's a nurse, she can help," were the words that were coming from the mouth of a woman whom I barely knew. The only introduction that I was given, to this woman who I had never met, was a push forward. I introduced myself, told her that I was a nurse, and offered my assistance.

She tried to assure everyone that she was just fine. As most mothers do, we don't want others to bother with us. I suggested she put some ice on her head at the site of impact. I knew that, minimally, she would have a goose egg on her head. She agreed and reluctantly started descending the bleachers to get some ice. Just as she stepped off of the bleachers, she lost her balance. The startled look in her eyes influenced my next actions. We, her friend and I, coerced her to go to the clubhouse and sit down on the couch for a few minutes. She didn't object now, as the pain was suddenly increasing. We escorted her to the clubhouse and put ice on the area where we suspected a bump would be sprouting up soon. We sat with her for a few minutes, repeatedly being assured that she was fine, after each of our inquiries. We offered to call someone to drive her home, but she refused. We continued to sit and watch and it appeared that there were no affects of the conflict between the ball and her head, until suddenly she said, "I think I'm going to be sick."

Nausea is a key sign of head injury. Now I wasn't so sure that everything was as fine as she was trying to convince us. After grabbing for the garbage can, just in case she vomited, I stepped up my nursing assessment; now I became the nurse. I started asking more questions.

"How bad is the pain?" Still, she assured me that it wasn't bad.

"How many fingers am I holding up?" Two was the correct answer. She wasn't seeing double.

"Look at my eyes." Her eyes were following my movements without problems. Both of her pupils were equal in size; unequal pupil size is an indication of increased pressure in the brain.

"Squeeze my fingers." We do this to check for equal movement. Increased pressure on one side of the brain will result in weakness on the other side of the body.

I didn't see any overt signs of head injury. Subdural hematoma, a blood clot in the brain, didn't seem apparent, but I knew that sometimes a head injury can result in bleeding and the symptoms may not be apparent initially. The bleeding may increase slowly and the symptoms will not occur until later. I see head injuries in the ICU and most of them come to us after a surgical removal of the hematoma that had caused neurological changes. I couldn't be sure that this mom wasn't experiencing some bleeding as we sat on that couch with ice on her head and a pail in her hand.

The nausea was the deciding factor that made me turn in a different direction. Instead of agreeing with her that nothing was wrong, I explained my concerns. The risk of the blunt injury causing a hematoma, and the risk that she may feel fine at that moment but suddenly lose consciousness in a few hours, was enough for me to be concerned. I told her that I thought she needed to go to the emergency room to be examined by a physician. I though she may even need to have a CT scan to be sure there was no bleeding in her brain. Every time she objected, I became more forceful.

"I'll be fine." She tried to convince me. I probably would have said the same thing, if I were in her place. But I wasn't going to allow her to refuse treatment. I knew what could happen with a sudden impact injury and I needed to encourage her to do the right thing.

Additional explanation that the ball could have caused a blood vessel to break in her brain was needed. I explained that the blood would spill out into her brain. There is not enough space within the skull for any extra fluid or blood. If a blood vessel breaks and blood leaks into the brain, pressure builds up inside the head and neurological changes occur. She needed to go the emergency room and have a doctor determine if this might have occurred.

It was that explanation that made her realize that I was concerned about her condition. It was then that she called her husband to come and drive her to the hospital. Someone would make sure that her son got home safely; all she needed to do was take care of herself. She went to the emergency room, probably spent several hours in the waiting room, because of the typical congestion on a Saturday afternoon. Later I discovered the physician had determined that she did not suffer from any internal head injury, and she was sent home with instructions to monitor her symptoms for concussion. Concussion is a mild head injury as a result of a blow, but no internal bleeding in the brain. Just as she was trying to tell me, she was fine. But, I felt better knowing that I did the right thing. If I had not sent her to the hospital and she had developed complications later, I would have had to deal with the guilt of making the wrong decision. It's better to err on the side of caution, especially when dealing with people and lives.

* * *

Not only do friends push nurses to the front of the crowd, so do family members. Riding home on the commuter train, after watching a local professional baseball game, my father, my son, and I came upon some commotion on the loading platform. As we walked past a crowd of people, we noticed a man on the ground. Another man kneeling beside him was obviously distressed, looking up into the crowd as everyone simply stood over him, doing nothing. It didn't take long to see that the man, lying on the train platform, was dead. His lifeless body, his pale face, his blue lips were all signs of death.

My father instinctively offered my help. "She's a nurse, she can help." Once again I was hearing those familiar words. My own father was pushing me toward the front of the onlookers. As I moved closer, I heard one of the spectators tell another he had just seen the man collapse. That gave me some information I needed. This man had just fallen to the ground. Maybe I could help him. My father knew I could; he had confidence in his daughter, the nurse. How could I let him down?

Two "Good Samaritan" strangers approached the victim at the same time. Each of us immediately knelt down on opposite sides of that lifeless body. As our eyes met, we could see that the other also knew what to do. We, two ordinary citizens, started working to save a life.

After establishing that this man had not suffered from trauma, but had suddenly collapsed to the ground, I hyper-extended his head to open his airway. He was not breathing. Now what? I had to make a decision. Was I going to perform mouth-to-mouth recessitation on a stranger who I didn't know? I had no idea if this person had AIDS, hepatitis, or any other communicable diseases. No, I decided that I would not place my mouth on his. I would hold his head, hyper-extended, to maintain an open airway. I moved a free hand to his neck. I held my fingers on the side of his throat, waiting to feel a pulse. As I continued to wait and search for a pulse, signs of a heartbeat, my partner whom I also had never met, was positioning himself over the chest. He was waiting for me to signal for him to start chest compressions. As soon as I assured him that there was no pulse, he started chest compressions. The two of us worked together until emergency personnel arrived on the scene. Emergency medical technicians, or paramedics, relieved us of our duty. We started early CPR but were no longer needed. Those who are trained for these public situations were there to assume care of this victim.

The crowd was dispersed and everyone went to their respective trains. All the bystanders were now on their way to their next journey in life, while the medical personnel worked to save another life. The train ride was not long, but it was just long enough for my father to brag about his daughter who had just saved the life of a stranger. Whether my father's favorite professional baseball team won or lost was not an issue now, his daughter, the nurse, was a hero.

✳ ✳ ✳

That was not the only time I was a hero in my father's eyes. I often become the hero when I intervene with my mother. My mom, who has chronic illnesses, never wants to be a burden to anyone. She lives daily with aches and pains and discomforts as a result of her ongoing illnesses. She has lived longer than any of her doctors would have predicted. But Mom continues to defy their predictions and continues to enjoy her life with her family.

Occasionally, when Mom is not her normal self, Dad will ask her if she is sick. Of course, Mom will deny that she is anything but perfect. Dad can see that she is not well, but she will not admit it. Occasionally, Mom will actually be undeniably ill but will not admit that she is as sick as Dad thinks she is. The two of them have been together since they were kids. They know each other well, but they continue to play the game. She claims to be fine; he knows she's not. She denies feeling bad; he knows she's sick, and worries. That is where I come in. I will be called on to provide the swing vote. I must decide if she is really sick or not. Often I have to cast the deciding vote for whether or not she seeks additional medical attention. But, in order to obtain my swing vote, we have to play another game.

I receive a phone call from my dad. "Hello"

A quiet voice starts on the other end. "Are you busy?" he calmly inquires.

"No, why?" seeking more information.

"Well, I thought if you were going to be out, you might stop by. Mom doesn't seem right, but she won't admit it." Then he goes on to give me the details of his assessment and what is worrying him. All of the conversation is carried out in a very low tone.

Suspiciously I ask, "Are you in the bedroom?"

"No, I'm in the garage." And Mom of course is in the family room on the other side of the house.

"I'll be right over." I assure him. And now I know that I must coincidently "drop in" on my way to whatever location I make up on that day. I assess the situation, sometimes scold my mother for not being forthcoming, sometimes reassure my father for worrying too much, but always I provide my expert opinion, the support they need, and the reassurance that I will be there for anything at anytime, day or night.

* * *

Sometimes I have to be the hero because I have been pushed to the front of the crowd. Sometimes I am reluctant to impose my nursing knowledge and skills on others, but feel obligated to help. But most of the time, I help because it is my natural instinct to help others in need. Most of the time, I help just because I want to.

One day I was at work and one of our family friends was in "my ICU." This is usually a difficult situation, when someone I know personally is dying in the ICU. It is hard to provide my friends with the support they need, while continuing to care for my own patients. And, it is never a good idea to be the nurse assigned to a friend or family member, because objectivity is compromised when the nurse is emotionally involved with the patient.

On this day I was, once again, the charge nurse. This allowed me to provide the emotional support to the family members, just as I was accustomed to providing support to nurses, doctors, and other family members when I'm in charge. But on this day, I tried to stay especially close to the bed that was occupied by my father's close friend.

Alex had been sick for many months. His family was aware that his condition was eventually going to result in his death. But Alex had bounced back from several events in the previous months and everyone was hoping that he could again. But today it became apparent that he was not going to make a comeback. His condition had deteriorated over the past few days and today the family had been called to his bedside because his breathing had suddenly become more labored. Alex had already made his end-of-life wishes known to his family and his physician. Alex was a DNR, do-not-resuscitate, so we would not do CPR if his heart stopped, but we would continue to provide comfort care, as long as he would need it.

Ginny was assigned to care for Alex on this day. She was providing the best care she could. But despite all her efforts, Alex was losing his battle with life. Respiratory distress was the only intuitive sign that Ginny had from him that told her that his time was near. His heart rate was normal, his blood pressure was normal, his neurological responsiveness had not changed, but Ginny had a feeling that Alex needed his family to come and be by his side.

As his wife, his two daughters, and his two sons gathered, they started asking questions. Since I was a familiar face, they seemed to gravitate toward me for their answers. I was not the nurse assigned to care for Alex, but the family quickly pulled me to the front of the crowd, once again. They were looking for answers and they wanted them from me because I was not just a nurse, but also a friend.

"What will happen now?" was the common theme of all the questions. They were looking to me for answers and reassurance to help them through this difficult time. I tried to answer the best I could. "As his oxygen level drops, the heart muscle will not receive the oxygen it needs and the heart will slow down and eventually stop." The one question that I could not answer was "When?" or "How long?" No one could answer that.

Throughout the day, I tried to stay as close as I could to the family, while continuing the rest of my duties. I had to leave the room during the prayers with the priest, because it was too hard to do my job with tears in my eyes.

Then as night fell, it was time for my shift to end. I had just spent twelve busy hours maintaining control over the entire ICU and the one room where my friends were depending on me. Now it was time for me to go home. Go home, take off my shoes, relax with my family and forget about my stressful day. But today, I didn't want to stop being a nurse at the end of the day. I wanted to continue doing what I do best. I needed to stay with my friends; they needed me there. They needed me to continue to answer their questions, to explain the minute changes as Alex slipped slowly towards a peaceful death. I needed to continue the care and support I had provided while on duty. Tonight, I was pushing myself to the front of the crowd. Tonight I needed to be a nurse off-duty. It was something that I wanted to do.

When my shift was over, I reported to the charge nurse of the next shift. I finished with my paperwork and returned to Alex's room. His family had been keeping vigil for over eight hours now. Several family members started to say good-bye and I informed them that I was not leaving.

"But, you are off duty," Janet, the daughter, tried to remind me.

"Yes, I am, but I think I'll just stay for a while," I could see the relief in her eyes.

As Alex slowly drifted, and his breathing deteriorated, all of the family took turns sitting at his bedside. After eight long hours, Alex was still holding on. It had been less than a year since I had sat at my own mother-in-law's bed for over four hours waiting for her to pass peacefully. Alex's family had patiently waited for him to go for over eight hours already.

As I sat with Janet, we discussed many things, his illness, his character, and all of his good traits. I answered all the questions that I could, but the one question of "when?" I couldn't answer. Janet and I discussed some possible reasons for why Alex was hanging on. Some patients don't want to die when the family members are in the room. Some patients, it seems, wait until the family leaves to go home, then they die just a few minutes later. Perhaps Alex didn't want to die with family at the bedside. So, finally, late in the evening we decided that each of the family members would go into the room, one at a time, and have a few minutes alone with Alex. Each person talked with Alex, told him what they wanted him to hear for the last time and said their good-byes. After all the loved ones had had their personal time with Alex, he still hung on. Despite the lower oxygen level, he still hung on.

Several times Janet tried to assure me with her words that she would be fine. "It's late, you should go home?" But her eyes told me she was glad I was there.

What could I do to help this grieving family? What could I do to make this terribly long vigil more comfortable for the family? Hot tea? Reassuring words? It seemed that all of my nursing skills were of no help. Once again I talked to Janet. It was late at night and Alex hadn't had a bath since early morning hours. Sometimes, patients pass away after they have a bath. I don't know if anyone knows why, but many nurses will report that their patients hang on and hang on for hours, but after receiving a comforting bath, they suddenly pass.

This was our next step. I wanted desperately to help Alex in whatever way he needed, to go peacefully. I spoke to Chuck, the nurse who was caring for Alex on the night shift. "Chuck, can I help you give Alex a bath? Maybe he is waiting to be freshened up?"

Chuck agreed with me, and he was eager to accommodate my wishes and provide whatever care was needed to comfort Alex and his family. So, Chuck and I bathed him, changed his linens, cleaned his mouth, changed the dressings on his sores, and tucked him comfortably into his fresh hospital gown. As we finished the bath, the family returned to Alex's bedside.

Within minutes, his oxygen level was dropping. Followed by a drop in his heart rate. As the heart rate slowed, so did his respirations. Alex looked good; he was clean and fresh. With his entire family at his side, Alex was finally ready to leave them. And Alex had decided, now it was time to go. Go to that peaceful place beyond.

∗ ∗ ∗

On that day, I couldn't stop being a nurse at the end of my shift. I needed, for them and for me, to continue being a nurse and a friend. I chose to go to the front of that crowd on that night—to be a nurse all day and all night. I hope my presence was of some support for this family. I hope that seeing a familiar face, not just those of strangers, helped relieve some of the suffering they were experiencing.

For this, I will gladly be a nurse, day and night. I don't want to only be a nurse when I am at work and receiving pay for my duties. I will gladly be a nurse any time of any day if it means I will make a difference in a life. Whether for a friend, for my family, or for a complete stranger, my goal is to save lives and make a difference. That is why I became a nurse. That is why I will continue to oblige those who request my assistance, those who push me to the front of the crowd, those who ask loudly for my help, those who just look like they need some support, and those who discreetly call, any day and any night.

CHAPTER 16

Beyond The ICU

The multiple ways the ICU nurse supports
others throughout the hospital.

The ICU charge nurse is the one who takes responsibility on any specific day to oversee the entire unit. She makes the assignments at the beginning of the shift. She decides which nurse will care for which patient, based on the needs of the patients and the competencies of the nurse. She makes rounds at the beginning of the shift, reviews the plan of care for each patient with the bedside nurse, and discusses any special needs for each patient. Throughout the shift, she assures that all the appropriate interventions are carried out. The charge nurse constantly monitors the state of the unit to assure everything is stable. At the end of the shift, she reports the status of every patient in the unit to the new charge nurse.

During her shift, the charge nurse provides clinical support to all the other nurses. She is at the bedside when any patient is "crashing." Crashing is the buzzword the nurses use when their patient is not responding to the treatment and the patient is deteriorating rapidly. The charge nurse is at the bedside for every Code Blue, every patient complaint, and every nurse request. Physicians call upon the charge nurse to discuss problems and also to discuss any special plan of care for their patients. She is called on to intervene with family members and visitors when they have a complaint, and occasionally to hear a compliment. The nurses, all twelve to fifteen of them, call her at various times of the day, when they need her support and help. The charge nurse triages the stable patients out of the unit and assigns all incoming, more critical patients to the appropriate bed location and to the appropriate nurse. The ICU charge nurse does many things and supports many roles throughout the ICU.

Not only does the ICU charge nurse act as a support within her unit, she also is a resource throughout the entire hospital. Because of the additional expertise the ICU charge nurse possesses, she is called to perform many duties that require advanced skills and critical thinking.

Throughout the hospital, there are a variety of patients and a variety of nurses. Each patient has different needs and each nurse has different abilities and confidence. The newer nurses have less confidence and require more support than the more experienced nurses. Charge nurses, on every floor, are usually one of the most experienced nurses on that unit. The ICU charge nurse is one of the most experienced nurses in one of the most demanding and most critical areas of the hospital. Throughout the hospital, at various times of the day, a variety of events occur when the nurse caring for a patient seeks the support of her charge nurse. If the charge nurse on that floor is uncomfortable with the situation, she will call the ICU charge nurse for support. The ICU charge nurse, over the years, has become the unofficial support person for the other charge nurses throughout the hospital. In addition to supporting her own unit, the ICU charge nurse also supports any other, less confident charge nurse who asks for her help.

Sometimes the nurses on the medical floor need more than a phone consultation from the ICU charge nurse. Sometimes the nurse on the floor needs the ICU charge nurse to come and assess a patient and provide her expert opinion. She needs help with a patient who is "crashing" on her unit. The Rapid Response Team was developed for this purpose. The Rapid Response Team is activated for urgent situations when any nurse needs assistance with a clinical situation that requires a higher level of support. The Rapid Response Team consists of the ICU charge nurse and a respiratory therapist. The ICU charge nurse is a crucial part of this team because she brings additional expertise to the bedside.

* * *

"I don't feel comfortable" is usually the first words out of the mouth of the medical floor nurse when the ICU charge nurse arrives. Samariah was an eighty-year-old man who had a blood pressure of 82/54. I arrived in the room to see he had already been placed in trendelenburg position and had an intravenous infusion of fluids dripping at a rapid rate. Trendelenburg position is when the bed is flat and the head of the bed is positioned lower than the foot of the bed. The patient who has a low blood pressure may be placed with his head lower than his legs in order to encourage what little circulation he has to go to his head and his brain. It is felt that gravity will promote the blood to flow to the lowest part of the body. If the head is lower than the feet, the blood flow will move in that direction and the brain will not lack any needed oxygen.

The nurse told me that before she activated the Rapid Response Team, she had already phoned the doctor and told him of the low blood pressure, which at that time, was 78/50. She was concerned that the doctor was not as worried about this low blood pressure as she was. He told her to give the patient five hundred milliliters of fluids, but did not respond with the same amount of distress that she was feeling about her patient's condition. The charge nurse, who was also at the bedside, provided additional information. This same patient was hypotensive a few days ago and the doctor was informed but he wasn't concerned at that time either. I immediately started asking questions in order to assess the situation. "What's wrong with this patient?" "Why did he come to the hospital initially?" followed by "What do you think is happening?" All these were addressed to the nurse caring for the patient. We had a discussion and I found

out the patient had renal failure and was admitted because his electrolytes were out of balance. He had not been eating well lately and
had, over the past few days, become more and more lethargic, sleeping more during the day than before. As I assessed the patient, we
reviewed his morning lab values and his intake and output totals for
the previous few days.

We continued, the nurse and I, to discuss what we thought was
happening. His skin was dry, his intake was poor, and he rarely
urinated. We decided that perhaps this patient was dehydrated and
could use some additional fluids. As we reviewed and discussed all
of the pertinent information about the patient, the intravenous fluids infused. After half of the prescribed fluid bolus—two hundred
and fifty milliliters—the patient's blood pressure was already 110/
62. It seemed that he needed that extra fluid to support his circulation. The situation was quickly under control. The nurse was comfortable with the patient's condition and was content
trouble-shooting this episode with me because of my comfort in the
situation and my ease throughout the entire event.

I suggested she call the doctor and ask if he wanted to continue
some intravenous fluids for this patient. Her response to my request
was a request of her own.

"Will you please call the doctor? He will listen to you more than
he will listen to me because you are an ICU nurse." It saddened me
to think that doctors don't listen to all nurses with the same sense of
confidence. But she was probably correct—that doctor might take
my input more seriously because I had responded to the Rapid Response call; I was the ICU charge nurse who dealt with the more
critical patients on a daily basis.

I phoned the doctor and told him what we had done, how the
patient responded, and what I thought. He informed me that he was
not concerned if this patient's blood pressure dropped. I suggested
that the patient might benefit from some fluids and he objected.

"Tell the nurses not to call me, I know this patient's blood pressure drops now and then and I don't care." This was all he initially

wanted to say. But I knew, if I let this doctor off the phone without more concrete instructions, the nurses on this floor would be uncomfortable and call him again and again, each time the blood pressure dropped below a normal level.

"Doctor, you know that these nurses are not comfortable with a blood pressure that low and they will call you every time Samariah's pressure drops. Do you want to give me some kind of order, something they can do when his blood pressure drops that low again?"

"O.K." he was responding under duress "Give him a five hundred milliliter fluid bolus of normal saline PRN BP less than 80."

"He only required two hundred and fifty milliliters to bring his blood pressure up this time." I reminded him.

"O.K. two hundred and fifty milliliters will be fine. But don't call me." Before he could hang up the phone, I repeated the order to him and thanked him for his time.

As I ended the phone call, the nurse was on my elbow listening to my conversation with the doctor. "Thank you so much. I wouldn't have known what to do if he just told me not to call." she said with eye wide open.

"Well, now you have a PRN order and you can treat the blood pressure when it drops." Before I returned to my unit I made sure both the bedside nurse and the charge nurse were comfortable with the patient's current condition and were comfortable with the outcome of the situation. They both assured me they were satisfied and thanked me for my time and help.

* * *

A week later, I was once again summoned to the medical floor by the Rapid Response phone. When I received the call from the nurse, Eleanor, she told me that she was caring for a patient who was having chest pain. She had already given her Nitroglycerin tablets under her tongue three times and one dose of Morphine. Usually chest pain will respond to either Nitroglycerin or Morphine, but this time the patient was still complaining.

"I'll be right there," I assured her.

As I entered the room, I saw a small elderly woman, Francesca. I was informed that Francesca did not speak any English—she only spoke Spanish.

"Anyone here speak Spanish?" I inquired as I gazed around the room at Eleanor and the charge nurse, both Filipino. Both of the heads shook from side to side. As I approached the bed, I saw a woman who was in significant distress. She was thrashing from side to side, each shoulder alternatively resting on the respective sides of the bed. Her face was pale despite the oxygen that was provided for her comfort.

Before I could ask any questions to assess the situation, Eleanor started telling me what she thought I needed to know. The patient was admitted for chest pain yesterday. She had a history of coronary artery bypass surgery many years ago and recently started having chest pains. An angiogram had showed that her coronary vessels were not occluded, but now she was admitted because of the continued chest pains. Her pain started about fifteen minutes ago and was not relieved by the Nitroglycerine or the Morphine. Eleanor had already paged the doctor but he had not phoned back yet. With all of that information, she looked at me as if to say, "tell me what to do."

I started looking at the entire situation. History of coronary artery disease, chest pain unrelieved by medications, oxygen is on. I quickly paged through the chart to see if there was any bits of information Eleanor left out.

"I don't see this morning's EKG in the chart." It was still early, I wondered if the EKG had been done. If it was in the chart, I could at least compare it to the previous one and see if there were any changes.

I am not an expert at interpreting EKG's but I will be able to see if there are any significant changes. We could fax it to the doctor when he calls back.

"EKG tech is on her way. I just called them too." She interrupted my thoughts.

I reached out for the patient's hand. As I held her hand gently, I resorted to my limited Spanish. *"¿Hablo Ingles senora?"* (Speak English Mrs?)

Her head shook from side to side.

"¿Dolor aqui?" (Pain here?) and I put my other hand on her chest.

Now she nodded affirmative.

"¿Grande dolor or poco dolor?" (Big pain or little pain?)

With that, she started speaking Spanish and rubbing her throat, as she continued to look around the room for help.

She was saying something about "la casa" and I knew that was her house, but I had no idea what she was trying to tell me about her house. All I could say was *"No comprende Senora."* (I don't understand, Ma'am)

While I was having this brief conversation, Eleanor was discussing the events with the doctor. His orders were to give her an anti-anxiety medication. He felt she was anxious and a small dose of that medication would help to solve her problem.

"She's very uncomfortable, are you sure you don't want to send her to ICU?" the nurse pleaded on the phone.

His response was, "No, just give the anti-anxiety medication and she will be fine."

Eleanor was not comfortable with that, but she had me there. For now I would have to bring the ICU to her. That meant that I would stay there at the bedside, I would provide the one-on-one nursing care, and I would stay with the patient until she was stable. And I would give the nurse the support that she was depending on while dealing with this unstable situation.

Within minutes, the EKG technician was at the bedside. The EKG was done and we compared it to the one of the previous day. There seemed to be no significant changes. As soon as the EKG was done, the nurse gave the anti-anxiety medication in the patient's intravenous line and the charge nurse was on the phone to call the patient's daughter at home.

The charge nurse explained to the daughter that her mother was having chest pain and we had given some medication. She talked briefly to Francesca's daughter, explaining the situation, and asked for her help. She needed to know if the pain was better or gone, and why her mother kept rubbing her neck. The charge nurse asked the daughter to speak to her mother, over the phone and interpret for us what she was so desperately trying to convey. While on the phone, the patient and her daughter spoke in their familiar dialect. The patient told her daughter that the chest pain was just like she had experienced at home, and she reported that the pain was getting better, but not gone yet.

She also told her daughter that she was rubbing her throat because her throat was dry and she was thirsty. After all of our questions were answered, over the phone, we gave Francesca a drink of water to relieve her thirst and dry throat, continued to hold her hand, and within minutes of the injection the patient became less and less restless and appeared to be calming down.

I resorted, once again, to my limited Spanish *"Senora, ¿Dolor grande or poco?"* (Ma'am, pain big or small?)

This time she shook her hand side to side as if to say "no" and she looked up at me and said *"muy bien."* I know that meant "very good," in other words—it's fine.

"¿ No Dolor?" (no pain?) I confirmed

"No" she assured me as she rested her head down peacefully on the pillow.

As the patient relaxed, Eleanor and I discussed the entire situation once again. We surmised that the pain must have been what the patient had been having at home and as the pain started, she became anxious and the anxiety seemed to be causing most of her discomfort.

At first we weren't sure that the anti-anxiety medication, ordered by the doctor, was going to be the solution. But we soon realized that he obviously knew his patient, and what was best for her, better than we did.

We discussed a plan for future episodes of chest pain for this patient. We jokingly suggested that the patient would need Nitroglycerine PRN chest pain, with an anti-anxiety medication as a chaser.

The situation was under control. The patient was calm and feeling better and Eleanor was relieved that the episode was resolved. Before leaving the unit, I confirmed that both the bedside nurse and the charge nurse were comfortable.

That incident went well, I provided the support the nurses needed, stabilized the patient and there was no need for the patient to go to ICU. Without the support of the ICU charge nurse, the medical nurse might have felt that this situation was more than she could handle. That nurse could not spend a significant amount of undivided time with only one patient because her other patients would not receive the care they deserve. If I had not been there for them, they might have influenced the doctor to transfer that patient to the ICU because of the increased amount of time she was demanding. Once the patient had been transferred to ICU, she would have immediately stabilized and we would have been triaging her right back out of the unit. Providing the clinical support to the other nurses during times of crises not only allows for them to learn how to handle these uncertain situations, but it also helps build the competence and confidence of the other nurses and it helps to avoid unnecessary transfers to the ICU.

✳ ✳ ✳

Not all calls for the Rapid Response Team result in stabilizing the patient and leaving them on the medical floor. Another call came in one afternoon from the cardiac medical floor. The charge nurse of that floor called and told me one of her patients could use my help. That was probably the most vague request I had ever received: "Could use my help." What did that mean? Low blood pressure? Chest pain? Difficulty breathing? I would have to wait until I got there to find out. Luckily, I just happened to be on the same floor as the patient, at that very minute, when I received the call. Only moments had passed when I suddenly entered the room.

"Wow, you got here fast" was my greeting.

"I was just down the hall. What's going on?" I inquired.

Sharon, the bedside nurse, told me that Phillip's wife had come out in the hall to find her. The wife told her he had suddenly fallen asleep in the middle of their conversation. Now Phillip wasn't responding like he had been all day. Sharon continued to tell me that this gentleman has been very talkative all day, teasing her and joking with her and his family. Now she said, "Something is really wrong." Her eyes were like saucers and she was obviously scared.

This time, instead of asking the usual questions like "Why is he here?" And "what is wrong with him?" I turned immediately to the patient. I noticed his head was slumping toward one shoulder, his eyes were closed, and his breathing was irregular. As I called his name, his eyes opened and he lifted his head, looking off into the air above my head. He was not looking at the face that had just yelled his name; he was looking toward some unknown air space. Sharon was right, something was really wrong.

In my head, I was thinking, *this guy's had a stroke.* He certainly wasn't teasing and joking now. I continued with my assessment. Phillip would not squeeze my hands with his left hand. He would grip strongly with his right hand, but his left just lay, flaccid, on the bed. He would not move both his feet as instructed. Again, the right would cooperate while the left lay lazy on the mattress. I stroked the bottom of both feet causing a bilateral reaction; reflexes in both feet were intact. The involuntary actions were happening, but he could not tell the left side of his body to move.

"Open your eyes," I requested.

He looked up again into that mysterious space above my head.

"Talk to me," I commanded.

Nothing.

"Tell me your name." Yet another attempt to elicit some response.

Still nothing, Phillip could not look at me, he could not move his left side, he could not talk, and suddenly I realized that he was not breathing.

"Phillip, take a breath," I demanded in a loud voice. He obliged and inhaled deeply. Now he was breathing, and breathing rapidly, but in a short time Phillip stopped breathing once again. I watched his chest and I watched the second hand on my watch. I waited patiently for about fifteen seconds, and then finally another deep breath initiated another few bouts of rapid breathing. As I watched and monitored his respirations, I noticed that his breathing pattern was very irregular. He would breath fast and stop, then breath fast and stop, again and again. This is not good, I ascertained.

"What are we going to do?" Sharon, with her big eyes asked again.

"I think he's had a stroke." I used my nursing knowledge to make a medical diagnosis.

"I think so too," she agreed.

As the two of us agreed that Phillip most likely had just had a stroke, his wife and daughter entered the room. Now they were asking what was going on. I introduced myself as the ICU charge nurse and explained that I had been called to look at Phillip because of his change in condition. I told them that I believed that he might have just had a stroke. I explained to them that his sudden onset of one-sided weakness and his inability to speak was what was making me come to that conclusion. I continued to tell them that I was also concerned about his irregular breathing; his pauses in respirations were worrisome.

"What are we going to do?" they echoed Sharon's question.

I explained that Sharon had already called his doctor and when he called back, we would probably be transferring him to the ICU. I had barely spoken the words when the phone in the room rang, it was Phillip's doctor and he wanted to talk to me. I described to him what I had assessed, left side flaccid—no movement, aphasia—unable to talk, and Cheyne Stokes respirations—irregular breathing patterns. I suggested that we take Phillip for a CT scan of the head immediately and then into the ICU. He agreed with my preliminary diagnosis and my suggestion.

The family was listening to my conversation, and as soon as I hung up the phone I met their inquisitive looks. "I just spoke to his doctor. We're going to take him downstairs, get a CT scan and take him to the ICU where we can watch him closely."

I interrupted my conversation with the family to make another call. This time I called the x-ray department. I wanted to make sure that the scanner was empty and we could do this one STAT. As the family listened, I explained the situation to the technician and was granted approval to bring the patient down immediately—the room was clear.

More questioning eyes continued to gawk at me as I completed my phone conversation. The wife and daughter were patiently awaiting more information. "I'm concerned about his breathing. See how he stops breathing for a few seconds every now and then." I held my hand on his chest as they watched closely. "I will be going with him, I will stay with him in the x-ray department, because I'm worried that he might stop breathing. After the CT scan I will take him to the ICU."

As the orderlies helped Sharon prepare Phillip for transfer, the family asked me where they could wait. After clarifying that they had previously been in our ICU and establishing that they were familiar with the waiting area, I suggested they wait in the ICU waiting room.

After Phillip was placed on transportable oxygen and on a portable cardiac monitor I escorted him downstairs so Sharon could finish her paperwork. The two of us went to CT scan then quickly into the ICU. Shortly after handing Phillip off to the nurse awaiting his arrival, I received a phone call. Once again it was Sharon. "I just wanted to say thank you for what you did. You were fabulous; I would never have been able to survive that situation without you."

"Thank you," I tried to be gracious.

"No, really. You were great, I really appreciate your help," she continued.

Again, I thanked her for the compliment and assured her I was available anytime to help. I only did what comes naturally to me. I assessed and intervened according to my knowledge, my expertise and my confidence. That is what the medical nurses want when they call on the ICU charge nurse's support. That same level of knowledge and confidence is what the ICU charge nurse is trying to teach each of those nurses when she remains on the medical unit to support those nurses. Once again, the ICU charge nurse was of assistance to the rest of the nurses for clinical assistance, skill and confidence building, and emotional support.

✳ ✳ ✳

Not only is the ICU charge nurse called to emergency situations within the hospital, Rapid Responses, and Code Blues, she is also called to emergency events outside the hospital, throughout the campus. When an event happens in the parking lot, on the curb, in the near proximity to the hospital building, the ICU charge nurse also responds. The emergency situation outside the building is called an "Onsite Emergency." The difference in the names allows all interested persons to be aware of the location of the event.

When Onsite Emergency is announced, the ICU charge nurse, an orderly, and a security guard respond. It is the job of the nurse and the orderly to stabilize the situation while the security guard secures the area and calls for additional help as needed. The skills of the ICU nurse are once again challenged.

✳ ✳ ✳

"Onsite Emergency, front entrance of the hospital. Onsite Emergency, front entrance of the hospital." was announced over the public administration system. I was charge nurse on that day so I was assigned to respond. I hustled to the cupboard in ICU, reached for the AED and the BLS backpack. The AED is an automatic external defibrillator commonly used by paramedics and others when someone has a cardiac arrest. If the person is in a life-threatening heart rhythm, the AED can shock their heart back to a regular rhythm. The BLS (basic life support) backpack contains gloves, masks, airways, gauze bandages and a few items that may be needed in emergency situations. My supplies were thrown over my shoulder and I was on my way as I announced to whomever was listening that I was leaving the unit.

As I exited the front doors of the hospital, I saw a small group of people gathered near a bench. I moved closer and noticed a parking attendant standing behind the bench, arms extended, supporting the head of an unconscious man. As I approached the crowd, the security guard was dispersing the gathering of onlookers.

"What happened?" I initiated an explanation.

"I saw this man over here and he was sitting having a cigarette. But the next time I looked over his whole body was shaking. I ran over to check on him and he just kept shaking so I called for help." The parking attendant, with no medical background, was astute enough to grab for the man's head, hold it in his hands to keep it from banging against the back of the concrete bench. "All I could do was hold his head." He looked at me as if to say, "Was that O.K.?"

"Looks like you did the right thing." I assured him as I started to assess the situation. The gentleman, with his head still supported by the shaky hands of the attendant, was now slumped backwards over the back of the bench. His eyes closed, his face pale and his respirations noisy.

"Let's lie him down on the ground," I requested as I looked around to see who I could draft for help. The orderly, the parking attendant and a second security guard all moved into place without being asked. Each of us secured an extremity and with the head supported, we gently lowered him to the cold concrete.

As I was extending his head to open his airway, the orderly was opening the backpack. His tongue was falling back in this throat, interfering with his breathing. Instantly I was handed an airway. The airway, inserted into his mouth, would hold his tongue forward and allow air to pass unobstructed as he inhaled. Mr. X, this unknown person, looked as if he was sleeping but we were not going to allow him to snore. We wanted that airway open and clear. With the insertion of the airway, his respirations were now quiet and unlabored.

I shook him, to stimulate some reaction, but he was not waking. He seemed content to take a nap on the cold hard cement. His shaking had stopped, probably a seizure, but he was now in a post-seizure state. After a seizure, the irritated brain needs time to recover and return to its normal state. During that time, the victim remains in a sleepy state. Mr. X seemed to be in this post-seizure sleep state, but it didn't last long. Suddenly, he opened his eyes with a groggy look.

He realized that he was not sitting on the bench having a cigarette. He was flat on his back and there were too many people looking down at him. As he spit out that annoying airway, he lifted his head, looked around, and tried to assimilate what was happening around him.

"It's O.K." I tried to reassure him. "You're O.K." I repeated. "Just lie here a minute." As I was commanding him, he looked up at me with questions in his eyes. He was not verbalizing yet, but I could only imagine that he was wondering, "Where am I?" "What happened?" and "Who is that woman kneeling over me?"

"What's your name?" I inquired

No response, just a blank stare.

"Can you talk?" A pause was followed only by an affirmative nod of his head. He nodded "yes" but said nothing.

"What's your name?" I tried again.

"Robert," he whispered.

"Robert what?" I pursued.

"Robert Constantine."

"Do you have seizures?" I continued my interrogation.

A disconcerting look stimulated me to ask again. "Do you have seizures?"

"No." his contorted facial expressions told me he didn't know why I was asking.

"You've just had a seizure," I informed him. "We're going to take you to the emergency room so you can be checked by a doctor."

Robert continued to have limited verbal interactions, while he watched those around him scurry to gather the needed tools to provide him with the medical care he needed. He remained dazed, still unsure of what had been happening while he was unresponsive. A gurney arrived with an oxygen tank on the side. Narrow tubing was wrapped under his nose and around his ears to initiate oxygen therapy as he lay flat on the ground. His breathing was slowly returning to normal. After assuring that he could stand, the orderly and the security guard assisted him to his feet. A minor pivot allowed him to be in a position to sit on the gurney.

Slowly he became more aware of his surroundings. The blank look in his eyes had disappeared. He was now beginning to appear more alert. As we wheeled him through the front doors, down the hall and toward the emergency room, I was able to determine that he was here visiting his brother. We arrived in the emergency room and I reiterated to the physician the events of the last twenty minutes. As he assumed care of his new patient, I set out on a mission to find Robert's family.

First I looked in the computer for a patient with the same last name. Once locating the other Mr. Constantine, I phoned the charge nurse on that unit. I told her briefly of the incident and asked her if any other visitors were with her Mr. Constantine.

"Hold on, let me check." She put me on hold while she continued the investigation. "His wife is here, do you want me to send her to the emergency room?" she asked.

I agreed with her plan and returned to the room where the physician was now examining Robert. He was still a little dazed and not answering questions very thoroughly when I interrupted. "His brother is a patient upstairs. His brother's wife is on her way down."

The doctor continued his examination while saying, "Thanks, that will be great, I can't get any information out of this guy."

Before leaving, I addressed my attention to Robert. I tried, once again, to explain to him what was happening. "Your sister-in-law is coming. You're in the emergency room now. They'll take care of you here." A nod of his head told me he understood.

I gathered my Onsite Emergency backpack and returned to the ICU. I restocked the gloves and airway that we used, packed it up, and placed it in the cupboard awaiting the next call. Then, I returned to my duties as the ICU charge nurse.

* * *

Why does the ICU charge nurse have to do it all? Why does she have to respond to the Code Blue calls, the Rapid Response calls, and the Onsite Emergency calls? The answer is because that person, who may change day to day, is one of the most practiced nurses in the facility. That ICU charge nurse has the clinical skills and the critical thinking ability to process the most troubling situations that occur. She will arrive on the scene, assess the situation, and intervene according to her level of expertise. She is going to make decisions, she is going to initiate actions, and she is going to assure that every patient is cared for according to her high level of expectations. The experience that the ICU nurse gains by caring for the most critically ill patients allows her to function in any situation. Her high-level critical thinking and reasoning supports her ability to handle any medical situation.

Nursing is one of the most highly respected professions. People, the general public, look up to nurses. In the hospital setting, floor nurses, in general, look up to the ICU nurses, and the ICU nurses look up to the ICU charge nurse. We, the ICU nurses and charge nurses, should be proud that we have earned this respect. We should continue to work hard to maintain that respect. We have chosen a highly respected profession, and we have chosen to work in one of the hardest, most highly respected areas of the hospital. And we must continue to strive to be the best and to continue to maintain a high level of knowledge and skill that will continue to assist the others who want and need our help and support.

A Good Laugh

Several years ago, I read one of the advice columns in the newspaper. The writer didn't seem to be asking for advice, but complaining about nurses.

The writer's mother had recently been hospitalized. The mother had experienced a sudden change of condition and had a cardiac arrest. As the writer entered the ICU, she witnessed some nurses leaving her mother's room, laughing. The writer felt this was insensitive and uncaring of those nurses. The essence of her complaint was; how dare they laugh when she was going through a traumatic experience.

The response by the advice columnist was that the nurses should, of course, have been more aware of their surrounding's, but laughing was not a sign of insensitive and uncaring behavior. The nurses may have been laughing at something unrelated to that patient.

Remembering this column reminds me of a few things. While in the ICU, each of us should be aware of our surrounding and what is happening outside of our immediate area. We must be sensitive to others and what is happening in their space. We must be cautious about laughing and having a good time, if family members are grieving in the next cubicle.

But we cannot stop the laughter all together because we must all remember that we may be laughing in order to keep from crying; laughter seems to be more acceptable in public than crying. The stress of the ICU, day after day, requires some form of occasional stress relief.

The family members who are visiting their critically ill loved ones should not be too hard on the nurse who is trying to find her own way of stress relief. Yet the nurses should remember to be cognizant of who is around, and act according to the needs of all.

CHAPTER 17

The Open Heart

The excitement of the heart, and saving lives
after cardiac surgery.

Many years ago, when I was a new ICU nurse, I remember sitting in the report room, listening to the previous shift charge nurse give report, and learning one of my first vocabulary words related to "open heart" surgery. She was giving a brief report on all of the patients in the unit. One of the patients had just been admitted with chest pain. The charge nurse was concerned that he had recently had a cabbage and was now having chest pain. I didn't catch the date that the patient had his cabbage, but I did hear that he was very anxious about this episode of chest pain.

My thoughts, as I continued to listen, evolved around the premise that cabbage was a gassy vegetable, but why would the gas, as a result of the cabbage, cause chest pain, or indigestion so severe that anyone would require intensive care treatment? After report was finished, I tried to clarify what I had heard. I wanted to learn more so I could be a better ICU nurse. I asked a few questions to clarify my uncertainties. I still remember how the more experienced nurses laughed as they explained to me that she was referring to the fact that the patient had had a "CABG" not "cabbage."

* * *

Coronary artery bypass graft (CABG) is perhaps one of the most common types of cardiac surgery. Many people refer to CABG as open-heart surgery, even though this type of cardiac surgery doesn't actually require the surgeon to cut open the heart. CABG surgery is done by replacing the coronary arteries on the outside of the heart.

Chest pain and heart attacks occur when the small coronary arteries, which supply the cardiac muscle with blood, become blocked and the heart muscle no longer receives oxygen. Pain alerts the patient that something is wrong, really wrong. In addition to chest pain, EKG changes will occur that alert the medical personnel the heart muscle is not getting enough oxygen. If the heart muscle does not get enough oxygen, damage will occur and the muscle will die. The cardiac muscle does not regenerate; once it's dead, that area of the heart is no longer useful.

Several options are available to maintain the patency of coronary arteries. After tests and work-ups, it is sometimes necessary to replace the useless clogged arteries and sew in new blood vessels to carry the blood to the distal portion of the cardiac muscle. These new blood vessels are taken from various locations throughout the body, sometimes from the legs, sometimes from the arms, and sometimes from within the chest cavity. Even though it is commonly called "open heart" surgery, the surgeon doesn't actually have to open the heart, the surgery is done on the outside of the heart.

When our hospital started its open-heart program, all of the ICU nurses received specialized training. Some of us went to the local University Hospital for training. As the program expanded, many of us became more and more proficient in providing specialized care for these patients. Today, we simply call them our heart patients. It's not that all of our patients don't have hearts, but these patients are with us only because of their heart surgery.

In our hospital, the nurse who will be caring for the patient changes into scrubs and actually goes into the operating room (O.R.) to assume care of her patient before the patient physically gets to our unit. Over the years, we have tried several different options to provide the best care for our patients. By having the nurse go into the O.R, at the end of the case, just as the surgeon is finishing up, she can get a feel for the condition of the patient. The nurse goes to the head of the surgery table and first receives a report from the anesthesiologist. He has been maintaining the vital functions of the patient throughout the surgery. The anesthesiologist will inform the nurse of all the medications that are infusing, all of the vital signs, and the general condition of the patient. The nurse can visualize and monitor the patients' vital signs for a few minutes before having to assume care of the patient. After hearing from the anesthesiologist, the nurse will move around the operating room and hear report from the circulating nurse. The circulating nurse will give additional information about what surgery was performed, and any special needs of the patient. After gathering all the necessary information, observing the stability of the patient, the nurse assists with the transport of her patient to the unit. After arriving in the unit, she now becomes primary care provider to her patient.

Some of the nurses who were instrumental in developing the cardiac surgery program at our hospital have moved on to other adventures, relocated or retired. However, several of us are still in the same unit. Now, we are the mentors for the newer staff; we are the experienced leaders who provide support to the less experienced nurses. Some of us, more mature experienced nurses, have been providing this specialized care for our heart patients longer than some of the surgeons have been doing the surgery. We, because of our longevity, our comfort, and our confidence are the ones who must be the patient advocates. We watch out for anything that doesn't seem right, and we make it right, for the patient's best interest.

* * *

One Saturday afternoon, Candice was called to the operating room to pick up her CABG patient. She was preparing to assume care of her patient, when at the head of the operating room table, she noticed that the EKG on the cardiac monitor did not seem normal. As she looked carefully at the monitor, she noticed EKG changes that looked similar to changes that occur when a patient is having a heart attack. Candice consulted with the anesthesiologist about the EKG pattern and the two of them watched closely as the pattern quickly returned to normal.

"That was interesting. What caused those EKG changes?" Candice inquired.

"Probably just a small air bubble." The anesthesiologist explained. "That's nothing to worry about. It sometimes happens and as the heart gets going, it passes through and gets reabsorbed."

Nothing to worry about, but as Candice waited just a few minutes; the same changes were, once again, appearing on the EKG monitor.

"There they are again." She alerted the anesthesiologist.

"Hum" was his response this time. "Let's just watch and see. It will probably go away."

So as Candice continued doing what we do in the O.R., she continued to watch that EKG monitor that was making her uncomfortable. As the O.R. team was done with all of their intricate tasks, they started preparing the patient for transport to the ICU. Candice continued to watch that monitor. The EKG changes were not going away this time.

"Something's wrong. I don't like what I'm seeing on that monitor." She shared with the O.R. team. "Dr. Louis needs to know about this."

Candice was concerned that this O.R. team would not pay attention to her concerns. They were finishing up their Saturday case. Many of them were supposed to be off on this Saturday and were called in extra to do this emergency surgery. She sensed that they didn't want to hear about any potential problems that could delay this case any longer.

Candice's role was to go to the O.R, assure the patient was stable for transfer, and take the patient to the ICU. But today, she was not sure that the patient was ready for ICU. What she was seeing on that EKG monitor was the same changes the she had seen many times before when patients were having heart attacks. Those EKG changes were signs that the coronary arteries, or perhaps just one, were blocked and were not providing the oxygenated blood to the cardiac muscle. Candice was not sure that this patient was ready to go to the ICU.

Dr. Louis, the cardiac surgeon, had already left the O.R. suite; he was elsewhere in the hospital making rounds on his other patients. The circulating nurse assured Candice that she had informed him, over the phone, of the patient's EKG changes.

In the meantime, the anesthesiologist had called in another anesthesiologist to view the EKG tracing. He, too, suggested that the EKG changes would "settle down" and there was probably no reason the patient could not go to the ICU. But Candice, with her expert experience, felt something was not right. Her concern was perhaps one of the new vessels that had just been sewn to this patient's heart was not in place properly. Maybe one of the new vessels had a clot in it. Maybe one of them was pinched or kinked as it laid in its new location behind the heart. Whatever was causing the EKG changes was alerting Candice that this patient's heart was not receiving the oxygenated blood that it should. The whole purpose of CABG surgery was to revascularize the heart, to provide clean and opened arteries that would provide a way for oxygenated blood to reach all areas of the heart. There should be no reason why this patient was showing signs of cardiac ischemia. Candice was concerned that if the O.R. team transported this patient out of their area and into her area, she would be left with an unstable patient. If there was something wrong with one of this patient's new grafts, this was the place that it would be fixed, not in the ICU.

As the O.R. staff continued to ready the patient for transport, Candice quickly picked up the phone on the wall. She called me; I was the charge nurse on that day. She rapidly explained what she had been trying to convey to those in the O.R, but she felt they were not listening to her. She was concerned that this patient should not be moved because something was causing the EKG changes, and something was not right.

I agreed with Candice and her concerns. My concern was that Dr. Louis might not have been aware of the extent of the EKG changes. Small changes may be insignificant, but the changes she was describing were not insignificant. I suggested that she call Dr. Louis herself, ask him to return to the O.R. and actually see the EKG changes before she would agree to accept the patient and bring him back to our unit. She agreed to do just that and as she was hanging up the phone, I heard her command. "Call Dr. Louis and have him come look at these EKG changes before I will take the patient to ICU."

I went on with my duties, and in about ten minutes, Candice returned to the ICU, alone. She explained to me that when Dr. Louis returned to the O.R., he saw the EKG changes, and excused her from the room. He told her they would call when they were ready for her to return. We went on with the rest of our work and waited patiently for another call from the O.R. to summons Candice. After, what I considered an unusual amount of time, the call for Candice to return had not come. So, I initiated a call to them. The nurse at the desk answered the phone. I simply asked if she could tell me what was happening. She informed me that the O.R. team was still in the room and that they had opened the chest up, again.

Now Candice and I started speculating as to what could be happening. Maybe one of the grafts was kinked and he, the surgeon, will straighten it out, resecure it and be done. Maybe one of the grafts had a clot in it and he would have to unattach one end, remove the clot and reattach the graft. All of this was purely speculation on our part because we didn't know exactly what the surgeon found, and how exactly he would fix what he found. What we did know was that the longer the patient stayed in the O.R., the more it supported the fact that Candice knew what she was talking about, and there really was something wrong.

Three and a half hours later, Candice received a phone call from the O.R. It was not to ask her to come get her patient, but she was told to hold on because Dr. Louis wanted to talk to her.

As she waited for him to come to the phone, she grimaced and said, "I wonder why he wants to talk to me?"

"Candice, what did you think you were doing?" He asked quickly.

Her eyes told me that she thought she was in trouble. "What do you mean?" she asked cautiously.

"Thanks to you, I just had to spend three more hours in surgery." He still was not making it clear to her, why he was calling.

"And ..." She encouraged him to go on, still not knowing if he was going to yell at her for doing something wrong.

"I had to redo two of the grafts and add another one. A total of five bypasses." He informed her.

"Oh," a short pause and a smile were followed by, " I'll take that as a Thank You." Now she could relax, knowing that she was right. "Do you want me to come and get the patient now?" Her tone of voice told him that she would be happy to bring the patient to ICU now that she was sure he was stable and not having a heart attack.

"No, they're not quite ready for you. They'll call when they want you."

As she hung up the phone, she knew that she had done the right thing. Candice was standing up for what she knew was right. She used her knowledge and experience to assure that the patient was taken care of properly. Candice stood up to the others who seemingly wanted to push this patient into the next step when he has not ready. She was a patient advocate on that day, doing what was right for the patient, not what was easiest for others.

* * *

Cardiac surgery patients are an enjoyable group of patients to take care of. Often they are healthy, except for the clogged coronary arteries. These patients often come to the hospital for a prescheduled elective surgery, one that they have been able to plan. Because of this, many of these patients come out of the operating room, recover, and go upstairs to the medical cardiac floor within forty-eight hours. Working in the cardiac surgery unit is a rewarding place to work.

The ICU nurse thrives on excitement and the adrenaline rush we get after an emergency is handled effectively. Each time a cardiac surgery patient is rolled into the ICU, we experience that adrenaline rush. These patients have the potential to be stable one minute and unstable the next. They are demanding of undivided attention and nursing care during the first few hours of recovery. The nurse cannot be distracted during this period. She monitors every beat of the patient's heart; she titrates medication infusions that control the blood pressure and heart rate. She performs all of the intricate nursing responsibilities while anxiously waiting for the patient's own body to resume normal control.

Most cardiac surgery patients may be unstable for a short period of time following surgery. As they stabilize, they will be monitored closely throughout the night and when morning comes, they will be out of bed, sitting in a chair, eating a light breakfast. To see how these patients recover from minute-by-minute monitoring to walking and talking within twelve hours is a very rewarding experience for the nurses. The excitement of the immediate post-op period, followed by the satisfaction of seeing the progress, is what we thrive on and enjoy. That is why most of us continue to work in ICU day after day. Providing care for these patients and seeing how our hard work pays off is what nourishes the average ICU nurse.

Not all of the patients recover "by the book." Sometimes the patient doesn't get out of bed for breakfast the next morning. Whether because the patient is sicker, has more risk factors, or has had some unexpected complication during surgery, some patients don't follow the expected pathway after surgery.

* * *

Pat was a sixty-three-year-old woman who was admitted to our ICU after experiencing a heart attack. Pat had been having chest pains for several days before she finally decided to come to the emergency room. By the time Pat admitted that she was not able to continue enduring the chest pain, she had already suffered through a significantly large heart attack. The coronary artery that was blocked supplied the left side of Pat's heart. Now, that strong left ventricle was weakened and Pat was also weakened and in our ICU.

We cared for Pat while she recovered from her heart attack. Her weakened heart was failing. Her cardiac output, the strength of each heartbeat, was about thirty percent of what it should be. With medications, and a balloon pump, we were able to nurse Pat back to a point of stability. Intra-aortic balloon pump (IABP) is a cardiac assist machine. A balloon lays in the aortic artery. It inflates and deflates with each heartbeat. The synchronous inflation and deflation of the balloon helps to increase blood flow to the coronary arteries and takes the workload off the heart.

Pat's cardiologist had requested a cardiac surgeon to consult, and he, too, was following her care while she was in ICU. Diagnostic procedures told us that Pat had significant blockages in several other coronary arteries. These additional blockages would result in subsequent heart attacks if not fixed. Once stable, she needed to decide what the next medical intervention would be. Cardiac surgery was the best option for Pat. Because of her weakened heart, it was decided she would rest and recuperate in the ICU for a week or so before the surgery. An additional week of healing time would hopefully allow the damaged heart muscle to stabilize before another insult in the operating room.

A few days before surgery, Pat was weaned off of the mechanical cardiac support and the medication that were supporting her vital signs. Her spirits were picking up, as was her endurance. Her color was once again comparable to others and she no longer looked like her bed sheets. All indications pointed toward recovery and readiness for the much needed CABG.

On the day of surgery, Pat was in the operating room for over twelve hours. Six hours is usually long enough for this common bypass surgery. After eight or nine hours we usually start worrying and wondering what is causing the delay. By the time our patient is rolled into the ICU, after twelve hours in the operating room, we know that things did not go "well" in the surgical suite.

As Pat was presented to us in the ICU, we quickly realized what caused the delay. Pat's chest did not display the usual dressing that covers the normal incision. Pat had a sterile drape across her entire chest. Pat was once again on the mechanical cardiac support machine that had facilitated her recovery from her heart attack the previous week. A multitude of cardiac support medications were infusing through the IV pumps. The surgeon, looking exhausted and sweaty was at her side.

We quickly learned that because of her weakened heart, and the extended time that Pat was on the cardiac bypass machine, her heart had swelled in her chest. Each time the surgeon tried to pull the ribs closed to secure the sternum, Pat's heart would stop. The normal pressure that the chest cavity applied to Pat's engorged heart was more than it could tolerate at that time. After multiple attempts to close the chest, and subsequent cardiac massages to restart the ailing muscle, the surgeon decided to bring Pat to the ICU without closing her chest. Instead of wiring the sternum together, and suturing the skin closed, the surgeon packed the chest with sterile gauze and covered her chest with a sterile adhesive drape.

Pat remained with us for several weeks. Eventually her mechanical cardiac support device was removed, the support medications were once again weaned, and Pat was once again getting better. The only problem was, her chest was still open. Through her recovery, she unfortunately developed an infection. Treating her infection was now a priority. She survived the heart attack, she survived the extensively prolonged time in surgery, but now she was fighting to survive the infection that could jeopardize her life.

One winter day, Rhonda was caring for Pat. Rhonda was an excellent nurse, who had been caring for Pat for many of her days in the ICU. When it came time for Rhonda to do Pat's complicated dressing change, she summoned my assistance. The dressing change required two nurses to don sterile suits, remove the drape, remove the packing and replace moist sterile packing in Pat's open chest cavity.

As we were inventorying our supplies, gathering a few additional tools, and dressing into our sterile coverings, Rhonda shared some concerns with me.

"Pat doesn't seem the same today," she whispered.

"What do you mean?" I inquired

"I don't know," a short pause, followed by "Nothing specific, but she just doesn't seem right." Rhonda couldn't articulate any specific reason for her concerns. "Her blood pressure is lower," sigh, "her heart rate is just a tad below what it usually is," another pause, "but most of all, her affect just isn't what it usually is."

With this, I started probing. "How's her cardiac output? How's her intake and output? How are her lab results? How's her oxygen level?" All my questions were answered, and nothing was abnormal.

"It's probably nothing," Rhonda started admitting, "just a feeling."

As I entered the room, I could see what Rhonda was referring to. Pat was not her usual self. She looked sad today, even though she denied anything was wrong, she looked like something was bothering her. "I'm just tired today," was all that Pat would admit.

Rhonda and I tried to engage Pat into our conversation as we undressed the chest. Despite our efforts to pull her into our lighthearted discussion, Pat didn't want to participate. She didn't want to oblige us, she just wanted to lie there, still and quiet.

The usually happy, energetic, outgoing patient was not in that bed on that day. Despite her mood, we continued our chitchat in an effort to lift her spirits, as we went about our business of changing this complicated dressing. We talked about everything except what we would expect to see once the covers were removed from Pat's chest.

What I was expecting to see, as we took the large drape off the chest, was exactly what I had seen a few days earlier when helping with this same procedure. We would see a clean incision. The sternum, which the surgeon had cut in half, would be separated and resting on each side of the open space. As we removed the packing, we would see the pink heart, positioned deep within the open cavity, galloping on and on as if it didn't even care that human eyes were gazing down on it. I remember the first time I helped the surgeon with this dressing change; I was in awe of what I was witnessing. I was amazed that I was actually standing over this person, still alive, and watching her heart beat in her chest.

This was just one more example of the excitement that ICU nurses experience—the excitement of watching a beating heart, laying in that gaping space, while we went about our duties. I was actually looking forward to seeing that amazing event, once again.

On this day, my excitement was replaced by terror. As Rhonda and I removed the last gauze from Pat's chest cavity, we watched the heart beat. But this time, as we reached for the first replacement gauze, we watched the heart stop. That heart muscle that had provided entertainment while we watched it dance in her chest previously, was not dancing for us today.

Pat's heart didn't want to oblige us, it just wanted to lie there, still and quiet.

Rhonda and I both saw that last heart beat. Our first instinct was to look at each other, then look back into the chest cavity just to make sure we were seeing the same thing. After looking, first at each other, then back into the chest, we simultaneously looked up at the cardiac monitor. The flat line of the monitor confirmed what we didn't want to admit, that we had just seen this dancing heart stop.

A million thoughts were running through my head. My first thought was, *Oh no, what did we do?* Then all of the doubts came at once. *Did we pull the packing too forcefully? Did we do something wrong? Did we forget something? Should we have done something different?* Too many thoughts and doubts were flooding my mind, but I couldn't focus on that right now. We needed to interrupt what Pat's body was trying to do. Pat was not going to die; I was not ready for that.

We called a "Code Blue" and started going through the steps to save this life. Rhonda and I had done this many times. We were both experienced nurses; we knew just what to do.

"You bag her, I'll start CPR." Those words came out of my mouth just like they had hundreds of times. But this time, as soon as the words left my lips, I realized that I didn't know how I was going to do CPR.

CPR—cardio-pulmonary recessitation—something we do in ICU all the time. Place your hands on the sternum, compress the chest, and squeeze the heart between the sternum and the backbone. That is what we did time and again when the patient had no heart beat. But with wide eyes, I looked down into Pat's open chest cavity. There was no sternum where I could place my hands. There was no chest to compress. All I saw was a gaping hole with a lifeless organ lying absolutely still at the bottom of the hollow space. As Rhonda began squeezing the ambu-bag that was delivering oxygen to Pat's lungs, she looked up at me with eyes wider than mine as if to say, "*It's right there, you have to do it.*"

We both knew what Pat needed was for someone to reach into her chest and squeeze blood and life back into her heart, but at that moment, I had never been more scared in my entire life. Her heart laid there, waiting for me, no movement, no life, no sign that it was going to start dancing any time soon without some help.

I stood motionless, as I contemplated what I had seen on TV so many times while watching those medical drama shows. I had seen doctors perform internal cardiac massage. But, there were no doctors in this room. The heart just laid there at the bottom of her hollow chest. *Should I reach my hand into her gaping chest cavity, gently place my fingers around the soft delicate sack that was vital to survival? Could I grasp the heart as gently as possible, without damaging it?* The adrenaline was surging through my body and what I really wanted to do was to clutch that lifeless heart and wring the useless blood out of it as new blood spilled back in.

The thought of placing my hand into her chest, gently gripping her heart, made me remember just how delicate the heart is. *What was I going to do? Would I be so bold as to break the rules and perform internal cardiac massage? Can I do this? Is this a nursing function?*

Should I actually place my hand on her delicate heart? Pat's life was, literally, in my hands. It seemed like hours passed while I deliberated in my mind.

It wasn't hours, it was just moments until the code team invaded our sterile space. Each of the team members dressed in their sterile gowns, before we allowed them to enter the room. The emergency physician interrupted my mind-boggling debate and immediately assumed my position and initiated the internal cardiac massage. I gladly allowed him to perform the function that he had been taught to do. I would eagerly initiate any nursing function that I was more comfortable performing. We coded Pat, gave her resuscitative medications, performed internal cardiac massage for what seemed to be an eternity. Despite all our efforts, Pat's heart was not going to accommodate our efforts.

Her cardiologist, Dr. Curtis, was the deciding vote to stop the resuscitative efforts when he arrived. He conferred with the emergency physician and shared his feelings that Pat was not going to survive this illness. He explained that over the past few days, he had begun to give up hope for recovery for Pat, but he didn't think her demise would come so soon. We stopped our measures to prolong Pat's death, and allowed her to go to whatever place it is that she wanted to be.

Now that the excitement and the adrenaline had calmed down, I once again started questioning myself. "Did I do something wrong?" I needed to know if Pat's death was my fault. I repeated the sequence of events to Dr. Curtis, exactly what we did, in the exact order and with the exact details. "What did we do wrong?" I asked.

"Nothing," he said emphatically. He assured Rhonda and I that nothing we did caused this unfortunate event. He explained that Pat's heart had been getting weaker and weaker over the past few days and that the packing was providing physical support, like a girdle, that was needed for Pat. And, as soon as we removed the packing, just as we were instructed to do, the heart no longer had the artificial support and could not gather enough strength to pump. He continued to answer all of our questions and relieved us from any guilt feeling we might have tried to tie onto ourselves. After a significant debriefing, Rhonda and I were able to rest assured that our nursing care did not cause Pat's death.

* * *

Looking back on this incident, I reflect on two different things. First, just how precious a piece of muscle is. The heart muscle works day and night to keep us alive. We don't have to think about it, it just keeps on dancing for our entertainment. I remember how astonished I was the first time I peered into Pat's chest and witnessed her heart beating inside that empty cavity. It was an experience I would never forget. Then, in the end, Pat provided me with yet another experience I would never forget, the opportunity to literally hold her heart in my hand.

The second thing I brought away from this incident was a remembrance of the intuition that Rhonda tried to explain to me that day. Her intuition that something was not right with Pat was correct. There was not one thing that any of us could put our finger on, but something told Rhonda that everything was not right. Perhaps Pat knew that her death was soon to come, but didn't want to burden us. Perhaps Rhonda knew, subconsciously, but couldn't articulate any specifics, she just had a feeling, in her heart.

The open heart—Pat's heart was open, literally—Rhonda's heart was open, intuitively.

* * *

I once worked with a cardiac surgeon, who was sometimes grumpy. He would yell at the nurses when they didn't do what he wanted them to do. Some of the nurses, those who were unsure of themselves and their skills, would get upset when he would scream and yell. Others of us learned to look him in the eye and say, "Please don't yell at me, I'm trying to do what you have asked." A simple request, and a firm reminder would usually settle him down and we could once again work together.

That doctor was an excellent surgeon. When his patients didn't recover as he wanted, he took it personally. He would spend hours sitting at the bedside, watching the monitor, watching the minute-by-minute changes and relaying verbal orders to the nurse who would accommodate his wishes. Each one of his orders resulted in incremental improvements, some minor and some more significant. If the nurse was caring for his patient, and he was not at the bedside, she would simply pick up the phone and dial his cell phone directly for an immediate response. He would never leave his patients in the hands of anyone else. He did the surgery, he was the doctor, and he was responsible.

One day I was having a conversation with him about one of his spontaneous, often uncontrollable verbal outburst. He tried to explain the reason for his behavior. He explained that his outbursts were only a result of someone not doing what was right for his patient. He explained that while in the operating room, he had his patients' life in his hands; he literally held their heart in his hands. It was his job, to stop the heart, fix and repair it, and jump-start it again. If he did his job correctly, the patient would live; if he did not, the patient would die. He continued this obligation well after he was done with his technical job in the operating room. He was dedicated and made sure that his same level of responsibility was carried out throughout the patient's entire course of recovery. He tried to explain to me that after holding someone's heart in your hands, you become a little bothered and sometimes irritable and angry, when another person threatens your hard work.

I learned a lot from this doctor. Not only was he a great surgeon who really cared for each and every one of his patients, but also he cared about the nurses and taught them what they needed to know to be excellent care providers in his absence. He did this because he only wanted what was right for the patients.

Only now do I understand what he was talking about when he tried to explain what it feels like to have someone's life in your hands.

CHAPTER 18

Who Calls the Shots?

What happens when the doctor is not available?
What will the nurse do?

Many years ago, when in nursing school, I relied heavily on my instructor for support and advice. I would explain any dilemma I had and my instructor would often ask, "And what are you going to do?" The correct answer, most of the time, was "I'm going to call the doctor." That answer, simply to call the doctor, was sufficient when in nursing school, or even for the first few years in the profession. During my early years in nursing, I went from depending on my instructors, to depending on the doctors. When unsure of any situation, I'd call the doctors for advice. I'd tell him what I saw, and wait for him to tell me what to do. He would give me advice and orders, and I would do what he said. Simply calling the doctor was sufficient when I didn't know what to do.

As a nurse gains experience, she becomes less dependent on others and more dependent on her own knowledge and instincts. Through education and experience, she learns what is needed for each patient. The nurses and the doctors work closely together to meet all the needs of the patients. The physicians must provide twenty-four hour care for their patients, based on the information given to them by the nurse. On a daily basis, the nurse is at the bedside, caring for the patient eight to twelve hours each day. The physician may only be at the bedside for short visits, sometimes only ten to fifteen minutes. During that ten to fifteen minutes, the doctor and the nurse will share information and thoughts and make a plan of action for the remainder of the day. If the patient is unstable, most physicians will visit the bedside more often than once a day. During these visits, the two will confer and plan, and if additional communication is needed, they will consult again and again during multiple phone conversations throughout the day or night. During his absence, the doctor depends heavily on the information he receives from the nurse. Assessment skills, knowledge, and critical thinking gained through experience are of utmost importance for an ICU nurse, and it's those assets that provide the physician with the trust he must have in each nurse.

The trust relationship that the nurse and the doctor develop is a key factor to providing the best care for each patient. The doctor must trust the nurse to inform him and provide him with pertinent information when the condition of the patient changes. The nurse must trust that the doctor will work collaboratively, respect her input, and provide the best care for each patient. Finally, the trust between physician and nurse provides for a collaborative, successful relationship. They work together, trust each other, and depend on one another to save lives.

* * *

Martin was a fifty-one-year-old truck driver who had a cardiac arrest while driving his truck along the local highway. Luckily, Martin simply veered off the side of the road and into a ditch when he lost consciousness. Fortunately for Martin, another traveler witnessed the accident and phoned the local emergency number. Within minutes, emergency personnel were on site and resuscitating him.

Martin had been struggling to maintain life, comatose and unresponsive for twenty-four hours. The first day I cared for him, I worked hard all day to keep him alive through several recurring cardiac arrests, adding and titrating medications that were supporting his cardiac functions, and hoped for the best outcome. The second morning, upon returning to work, I was actually surprised to see his motionless body still lying in the bed. I couldn't believe that he had survived the twelve hours while I had been home comfortably in my warm bed. I had expected that the nurse who relieved me would continue fighting through the frequent cardiac arrests, until Martin's heart would no longer respond. Despite my expectations that he would not survive through the night, now I was seeing that his cardiac function and his blood pressure were almost normal, but unfortunately, his brain was giving us no signs of improvement.

As I listened to report and completed my assessment, I started planning my care. In addition to focusing on short-term goals, like preventing any further cardiac arrest, I would also have to start thinking about what Martin would need to get better. Each morning, after completing my assessment, I develop, what I call, my "shopping list"—a list of physician orders that I need. I keep this list handy so when the doctor makes rounds, we can discuss the status of the patient and decide on a plan for the day. The doctor will then write the orders.

This is a daily occurrence. The doctors and the nurses work closely together to assure all of the patients' needs are met. In order to be successful, the nurse needs to have her "shopping list" ready when the doctor makes his rounds.

I was glad to see Dr. Anders, the internal medicine specialist assigned to Martin's case, making early rounds on that day. I had accumulated a few shopping list items in my head already.

"How's he doing?" he asked in an open-ended request.

"His blood pressure is better, it's been staying above ninety systolic, but he's still on Levophed, Epinephrine, and Dopamine." Those medications were supporting his blood pressure, but Martin was not as dependent on them this morning as he was yesterday.

"Let's wean the Epinephrine, as long as his blood pressure stays above ninety," he muttered as he did his own assessment.

"When was the last time he had V-tach?" He was as eager as I had been to find out what time his irritable heart finally calmed down.

"None since about two in the morning." I was glad those life-threatening arrhythmias might have been obliterated with some of our medications.

As Dr. Anders continued with his assessment I persisted, "His fever spiked up to 103 early this morning. I placed ice packs in his armpits while I was waiting for you. Can we give him a Tylenol suppository?"

"Sure," he obliged my request.

"And his urine output's low," I continued, "he's getting a lot of fluids with all the IV's," I paused, waited a fraction of a minute then provided a suggestion, "he's not on any diuretic."

Again, he agreed with me. "Give him twenty milligrams of Lasix, and let me know how he responds."

"His eyes are dry, Can I get some artificial tears from the pharmacist?" These "tears" are a moisturizing and comforting measure that would probably make me feel better than it would Martin.

A nod of approval encouraged me to keep going as Dr. Anders reached for the chart and opened it to the section holding the physician order forms.

"He has good bowel sounds and his albumin level is low; shall we start some feedings?"

Another nod of approval, as he reached into his pocket, pulled out his pen and started writing, encouraged me to go on. I recapped our plan of care.

"OK, I'll wean the Epinephrine. If I get that off, I'll start with the Levophed but leave the Dopamine on for the urine output. I'll give him a suppository for his fever, diuretics, eye drops, insert a feeding tube and start feeding him."

As I spoke, he wrote down everything that was on my "shopping list."

As he closed the chart, I added, "Labs in the AM?"

He opened the chart for one more addition and closed it quickly. As he, once again, started to leave the bedside, I remembered one more thing so I quickly added my last request. "I'll have the dietitian come see him and give us her recommendation for maximum feeding needs." He again concurred with a nod of his head as he left the unit.

* * *

That is not an unusual scenario in the ICU. Nurses spend many hours daily assessing, evaluating, and intervening on behalf of their patients. Those same nurses collaborate daily with the doctors when they make their, often brief, daily rounds. Because we work side by side with the physicians while caring for their sickest patients, we learn. We continue to learn on a daily basis. We see a lot of patients, a lot of illnesses, and a lot of medical interventions. We see doctors come in to assess, diagnose, and treat these critically ill patients. After many years of ICU nursing, we often know what the doctors will plan, what they will order, and many times what they are thinking before they offer to share their thoughts with us. The nurses and the doctors are team members; they collaborate, and they depend on each other to provide the best care for their patient.

After the daily rounds, the nurse will carry out all of the physician's orders and the interventions that were discussed. Then, throughout the rest of the twenty-four hour period, when the nurse detects a change in the patient's condition, she will once again contact him and discuss the changes. She calls the doctor, consults, obtains an order, and carries out that order. Each of her actions is preceded by a specific order and every time the patient's condition changes, she calls the doctor again, obtains more orders and performs the next intervention.

This process works most of the time, but in the ICU, conditions can change so suddenly that it is often not possible to consult with the doctor each time the patient's condition changes. An ICU nurse often must initiate life-saving interventions and then inform the doctor after the fact.

Because the ICU is a different arena, and the patients are more likely unstable, the doctors depend on the nurse to provide the appropriate care in emergency situations based on some pre-approved guidelines. In the ICU, I've learned to depend, not only on the physician's advice and on these guidelines, but also on my own knowledge, experience, and gut feelings; the same knowledge, experience, and gut feelings on which the doctors depend.

Physicians depend on us to care for their patients when they are not there. They depend on us to provide the needed measures in a timely manner; they trust that we will provide the necessary care and they trust that we will do this instinctively and won't stop to call them before we save lives.

* * *

Joshua, a 63-year-old man, was transferred to our ICU after being admitted to the medical floor for complaints of difficulty breathing. Joshua was admitted with pulmonary edema, a condition that results in an accumulation of fluids in the lungs. The extra fluids will cause difficulty breathing, but can be treated with diuretics and oxygen in the early stages.

After spending a few hours on the medical floor, Joshua was becoming more and more short of breath. The nurses upstairs were communicating frequently with Dr. Young, but it soon became apparent that Joshua needed a higher level of care and was transferred to us.

As he rolled through the door, I saw a thin, frail, graying man who was sitting upright on the gurney. An oxygen mask was providing him with one hundred percent oxygen, as much as we could possibly give. But despite the oxygen and the diuretics that had already been given upstairs, Joshua was not getting better, and was quickly deteriorating.

We, the team of nurses in ICU, worked quickly to lift Joshua off the gurney and onto the bed. We attached him to our cardiac monitor, blood pressure cuff, oxygen sensor, and IV pump machine and within minutes, we were aware that this was not going to be a simple transfer. His respiratory rate was in the high forties, and his oxygen saturation was only 86%. It was obvious that he was struggling to breath and would soon tire out.

My first command was for the unit secretary to phone Dr Young. I knew that intubation and mechanical ventilation was what Joshua needed to save his life. If we didn't act soon, he would stop breathing and die. Within minutes, I asked again, "Did you call Dr. Young?" and I was informed that his answering service was paging him.

"Call him again." I shouted, now I was feeling anxious for Joshua, his breathing was becoming more and more shallow. I knew he was pooping out.

"Forget it." I snapped at the unit secretary, "Call the emergency doctor, tell him to come and intubate this guy." I could no longer wait for Dr. Young to respond. I had to act, based on what I knew had to happen and I could not delay treatment while waiting for a phone call that would allow me to tell the physician of his patient's condition and wait to hear the orders he would give to me. I needed to act on my own instincts and save this man's life. I would have to inform the doctor later.

Only minutes passed and we had Joshua sedated and intubated. Now he was breathing safely with the assistance of the ventilator. Dr. Young called back when we were in the room, performing our life saving procedure. The unit secretary informed him of what we were doing and he acknowledged that we had done the right thing and would come soon.

Dr. Young interrupted his office work and came immediately to the unit. He provided me with all the orders I needed to care for Joshua. As he was leaving to return to his office, we were thrown yet another curve ball. This time Joshua suddenly went into a life-threatening arrhythmia, ventricular tachycardia. The ventricles of the heart were not beating rhythmically as they usually do. They were ineffectively trying to contract more than one-hundred eighty times each minute. The heart cannot pump blood to the body with this ineffective heartbeat. His weak heart was put through too much stress during his respiratory distress, and now it, too, was pooping out.

"Code Blue," announced three times over the public administration system, alerted everyone that we were having a life-threatening emergency in the ICU. We successfully resuscitated Joshua, quickly defibrillating, shocking, him back into a regular rhythm. We started medications that would reduce the irritability of his heart that was causing his life-threatening arrhythmias. Now, only six hours after being admitted for what he thought was a cold, he was in the ICU teetering between life and death.

Dr. Young worked beside us as we stabilized Joshua. His cardiac rhythm, his blood pressure, and his breathing were all supported with medications and machines. We thought we had Joshua stabilized so Dr. Young returned to his office, the other nurses returned to their own patients, and I returned to my paperwork.

Within minutes, I heard the cardiac monitor alarm ringing. As I looked up, I saw the same ventricular tachycardia that had compromised Joshua earlier. I quickly activated the "Code Blue" team once again. We started CPR, we defibrillated him, and we gave him more medications. His heart quickly returned to its regular rhythm. After the second "Code Blue," I notified Dr. Young. I informed him of what I had done. He simply said, "Thank you, I'll stop by after office hours."

Despite all of my efforts to prevent recurring arrhythmias, Joshua continued to have frequent cardiac arrests. The repeated spontaneous bursts of his pulseless ventricular tachycardia were causing frequent bouts of commotion in the ICU. Each time I would push the Code Blue button, start CPR, give medications and as the code team arrived, I would use a team of staff to resuscitate him back to life. After the first few "Code Blues," I learned that what Joshua required most to restart his weak heart muscle was a rapid defibrillation. After the second or third "Code Blue" was initiated, I was into a routine, push the button, shock him, then turn the team away when they arrived because I had already completed the task at hand.

As I quickly learned what Joshua needed most was defibrillation, I was able to settle into a sequence. Because he was so frequently in and out of this deadly rhythm, I would not push the Code Blue button; I would not wait for the team to arrive; and I would not call the physician to inform him of each change before I provided the emergency care that was needed. I would simply proceed, again and again, to defibrillate Joshua back into his normal rhythm. I didn't have time to leave the bedside long enough to call the doctor to ask permission, or get physician orders to perform all the tasks that I was doing to save his life. I simply followed the ICU guidelines that provided me with permission to perform emergency care without waiting for directions. I would do what was needed, and I would inform the doctor later.

On this day, I sporadically communicated with the doctor, told him what was happening and he depended on me to provide the appropriate interventions, without his presence. He gave me orders to adjust the medications in order to get the desired effects that were needed. I worked hard all day trying to save Joshua. I defibrillated him more than a dozen times in the twelve hours that I worked. I shocked him; I gave medications; and I shocked him again, and adjusted more medications. Each time, my actions were based on what I knew was right for the patient. I did not wait for the doctor to give me instructions each and every time another interventions was required.

When caring for Joshua, I couldn't wait for his doctor to tell me what to do. I needed to act quickly, based on what I knew was right. I couldn't stop and call for orders or Joshua would have died. I couldn't wait for a physician to tell me that he needed to be intubated and later in the day, I couldn't call his doctor each time he needed to be defibrillated. I provided the care that his doctor trusted me to provide, and I kept him informed, after the fact.

* * *

Nurses learn from and depend on the doctors just as doctors depend on nurses and sometimes learn from them. An inexperienced nurse will naturally depend more on doctors and less on her instincts. An experienced nurse will still depend on doctors, but will rely equally on her own experience. In my early years, I depended on others to tell me what to do. Now, I tend to rely more on my experience when making critical decisions regarding patient care. Because of my years in the ICU, I can usually anticipate what the doctor will order before the orders are given. After many years in ICU, my frustration now generally stems from the occasional conflict arising when my experience tells me to take one course of action, but the doctor will not accommodate what I know is right.

* * *

Mary, an eighty-year-old woman, was transferred to the ICU from the medical floor. She had been admitted the previous day after experiencing a heart attack at home. Mary seemed to be doing fine during the night but this morning she suddenly became short of breath and started having more chest pain. Dr. Burns assessed her needs and determined she needed an intervention to open the vessel of her coronary artery. The procedure was uneventful and Mary was transferred to the ICU after the procedure. We were told that everything went well, but she needed to come to ICU just for observation because of her advanced age and her recent heart attack.

Upon arriving to the ICU, Mary was receiving oxygen through a mask. Her oxygen level was being monitored and was stable at ninety-four percent; anything over ninety-two percent is usually acceptable. She was awake and alert, slightly restless, and telling me that she was feeling "just fine." I settled Mary into her new surroundings and reviewed the post-procedure orders. As Mary's daughter joined her mother in the ICU, I explained the post procedure routine to both Mary and her daughter. My initial assessment provided me with some concerning information. Mary denied that she was having difficulty breathing, but I observed her respiratory pattern to be faster than normal. Her chest muscles were obviously assisting what should be unlabored breathing. I watched the oxygen level on the monitor closely, and decided to take the wait-and-see approach. I couldn't put my finger on anything specific, but I just had a feeling that something was not right.

Experienced nurses develop a different sixth sense—one that tells them when something is wrong. Sometimes we can't initially put our finger on the issue, but eventually whatever is wrong rises up and requires immediate attention. This was one of those situations, I couldn't quite figure it out, but my gut was telling me to watch Mary just a little bit closer.

I stayed close to Mary. I chatted with her, I chatted with her daughter, just to remain in the room until those uncomfortable feelings would be relieved. It wasn't long until my uncertainties developed into some concrete concerns. Mary's slightly restless activities quickly progressed to thrashing of her arms and legs. That lovely lady who was previously in an alert state of mind gradually turned into someone who didn't know where she was and why she didn't have her clothes on. Her breathing pattern, which she formerly denied was a problem, was obviously more labored now. Short of breath and confused, now I had something to substantiate my gut feelings.

I increased the oxygen level as her oxygen saturation level dipped below ninety. As I reassured her to try to alleviate her confusion, I completed a reassessment. Her lung sounds were no longer clear, now I was hearing some crackles, demonstration of fluid collection in her lungs, and less air movement throughout her lung fields. I called the respiratory therapist for reinforcements as I reviewed all of the physician orders once again. No respiratory treatments were ordered, no diuretic to clear the fluid, nothing that would help me reverse this distress for Mary. We had no orders to provide us tools to help, so I needed to call her doctor.

I placed the call. The answering service would page the doctor, "He'll call you right back." I was assured. As I waited, what seemed like an exorbitant amount of time for the physician to return my call, I continued to provide small efforts to help Mary.

I repositioned the head of the bed to help with her breathing. I reminded her over and over again of where she was in an attempt to orient her confused mind. I waited patiently but never received that call that I was waiting for. I called again and received the same person attending to the answering service phones. That anonymous person suggested that the doctor might actually be at my hospital. He would page him again, but in the meantime I would also ask that he be paged with the public administration system within the facility.

After the second attempt, I still received no response. Mary was slipping into that gray area; that area where I knew she was not right, but not yet in major distress. By now, I was tired of being patient, I knew what needed to be done, but the doctor was not there to do it. I tried one last option. I called directly into the procedure lab and asked if Dr. Burns was performing another procedure. The secretary who answered the phone informed me that he was "tied up." I was only allowed to speak to him through the interpretation of the nurse in that department. I relayed all of my assessment, the confusion, the difficulty breathing, and the new crackles in the lungs. We agreed to increase the oxygen level, give Mary a respiratory treatment to try opening up the air passageways in her lungs, and give some diuretics to get rid of some of the extra fluids that had been infused during the procedure. Often older patients will develop problems as a result of increased fluids during a procedure, and often a little extra attention is all that is needed to prevent further complications.

Within minutes, the respiratory treatment was completed and the diuretic was in her system. I continued to wait patiently for even the slightest change in her condition. As time passed, despite our efforts, there was no change. Once again I phoned Dr. Burns. This time I was told, "Don't worry, give her some time, she'll be fine." He was not hearing the desperation in my voice; he was not at the bedside to see what I was seeing. Despite my efforts to instill the urgency of this situation, Dr. Burns wasn't giving me what I wanted. I wanted attention to the respiratory status of this fragile eighty-year-old lady.

My first response was to doubt myself. "Maybe he is right, maybe

I'm overreacting, maybe I should wait and see," was going through my mind. I doubted myself, I tried to remind myself that the doctor did have more education, and he did have as much experience as I did. I'd have to give him the benefit of the doubt. But it wasn't long until those thoughts were gone again and I, once again, wanted some attention and interventions.

Mary was now significantly more short of breath and her confusion was not resolved with gentle words. Now she was panting inbetween her frequent requests to go home, and now was starting to cough, a moist cough that allowed me to hear the moisture in her airway. Another call to the doctor's location resulted in the secretary relaying the message that he was busy and could not come to the phone. She relayed a message that he would come see Mary when he was done with his procedure.

That was not good enough for me. I could not stand by and watch this cute little lady deteriorate if I could prevent it. Since the doctor was not able to come and assess the situation for himself, I had no choice but to take control and make sure that my patient got what I knew she needed.

I consulted with the charge nurse. Situations like this require alerting those higher in the chain of command. When something is not right, the charge nurse needs to know. Often the charge nurse can enlist the support of others, the nurse manager, the medical director, or whoever needs to be involved. Hopefully this would not get to that point, hopefully the doctor would be strolling in soon and we could resolve this issue. After consulting the charge nurse, she agreed with my plan of action. I was going to make one last phone call to the department where the doctor was in the middle of a procedure. I emphatically requested that the secretary relay my request for the orders that I knew Mary needed: arterial blood gasses (ABG's), chest x-ray, a catheter, and oxygen in any form that would maintain an adequate oxygen level. I couldn't wait for the doctor to come to my unit and see for himself; he was too busy. I needed to act now, and I needed to do what I knew this patient required. When I heard his approval in the background, I wasted no time implementing the stat orders that were not coming fast enough. I quickly got the ABG's that would allow me to evaluate Mary's oxygen level. While the portable x-ray was being taken, the ABG results were being processed. I inserted a catheter into her bladder in order to monitor her urine output from the diuretics. I requested all of these orders over the phone, because my gut was telling me, something was not right.

It didn't take long to obtain the stat results for the requested test. The ABG results showed that Mary had an extremely low oxygen level. The chest x-ray showed pulmonary edema was causing the shortness of breath, the drop in oxygen, and her frequent moist cough. Her lungs were filling up with fluids, extra fluids that she had received during her procedure. Her heart was old and weak and the extra fluids she had received during her procedure were just enough to tip her into this fragile respiratory state.

I once again increased the oxygen level; this time I placed Mary on a mask that would provide one-hundred percent oxygen. This was the most I could do on my own. I did, however, command the respiratory therapist to get the bi-pap ready so we could quickly secure to Mary's face if she continued to deteriorate. Once again, I tried to interrupt Dr. Burns in his procedure. Minutes seemed to pass like hours while I waited for his response. Once I finally was allowed to talk to him, I reiterated all of the facts, Mary's condition, and the results of the tests. This time he heard the distress in my voice. He was finally convinced that Mary was in trouble. This time, on the other end of the phone, I heard an almost frantic voice saying, "I'll be right there."

By the time he arrived in the ICU, I had the respiratory therapist nearby to assist with intubation. Mary had quickly moved beyond the bi-pap option and now was in need of imminent intubation. The tray was ready, the team was ready, and I was waiting impatiently for the overdue medical treatment. Mary had deteriorated significantly and it seemed like I was the only one who was helping her. She was going to need to have a breathing tube placed into her lungs. The support from a mechanical ventilator would help maintain life until we, her trusted medical team, could treat her through this episode of pulmonary edema.

Within minutes of arrival, the doctor had intubated Mary—she was breathing easier with the support of the ventilator. I was also breathing easier knowing that Mary was safe. After all the activities had settled, Dr. Burns asked me to again explain the sequence of events. After listening, this time attentively, to all of my assessments and all of my interventions, he apologized for not doing what he now knew was necessary before Mary deteriorated. He thanked me for taking control of the situation, doing what needed to be done, and rescuing both Mary and him.

* * *

The ICU nurses make life and death decisions regularly. Most decisions are supported with doctor's orders. The doctors and the nurses work together, collaboratively assessing, writing orders and carrying them out. Many of the doctors' orders require additional decision-making on the part of the nurse; titrate infusions based on blood pressure, titrate oxygen based on ABG results, medicate based on pain relief. The nurse constantly modifies her nursing care based on changing assessments and modifiable physician orders for specific interventions. Because of the nature of the ICU, the physicians will regularly write orders that require decision-making skills from the nurse. It is expected, in the ICU, that the nurse will make decisions based on the patients' changing conditions and notify the doctor if those decision-based interventions are not successful. ICU nurses are expected to have critical thinking and decision-making skills. The doctor gives the order; the nurse carries it out, based on her assessment of the patient, her knowledge and experience, and her better judgment. That is what is expected in the perfect scenario.

Sometimes that perfect scenario doesn't happen. Sometimes the physician orders do not provide the immediate interventions needed, and sometimes the orders do not include what is necessary for a patient's changing condition. In those cases, the nurse must use what orders she has, reassess the situation and call the doctor for additional measures. It's imperative that the nurse communicates with the doctor and the doctor provides the orders necessary for the changing conditions. However, occasionally, as with Joshua, the nurse must rely on approved guidelines. And with Mary, the nurse must be assertive to get the proper orders over the phone and must act emergently and without waiting for the doctor to arrive. The nurse must do the right thing, with or without the doctor present.

Why is it that the ICU nurse will take matters into her own hands? Why is it that she is bold enough to demand treatments and tests without waiting for the doctor to see the patient? Is it because she has been expected to make decisions related to the best care of the patients on a daily basis and she feels obligated to continue? Is it because she knows that the doctors have come to expect that she will do what is right, no matter what? Has her knowledge and confidence, that the physicians have learned to rely on, caused her to step out of her box and into his? Why is it that the ICU nurse is sometimes expected to do this?

Maybe, because of the close relationship the ICU nurse has with the doctors, or because of the daily collaboration and learning, she is more secure in her out of the box role that she plays in emergencies. Is the ICU nurse practicing medicine when she tells the doctor what to order based on what she knows is needed? Is that the right thing? When do we step over the line? When do we stop practicing nursing and start practicing medicine? It's not a problem if we do the right thing, but what is the right thing?

After working in the ICU for over twenty-five years, I have developed a comfort level with the doctors and myself. I have learned from many excellent physicians, and I have also learned from some less proficient ones. I have worked side by side, and have learned from the best. Often I feel like I'm the one calling the shots, but only when necessary and for the best interest of the patient, and always with the support of the physicians.

Undivided Attention

When caring for critically ill patients, the nurse must give them all of her undivided attention. One day when I went to work, I put the business card of my hairdresser in my pocket. I was meaning to call for an appointment for a haircut the next day. I really needed a haircut because I was long overdue. During the day, I totally forgot to make that call. I was so focused on my patients that my haircut didn't even enter my mind. The next day, on my day off, I phoned for an appointment. I made the appointment for the following Wednesday. But, on that same Wednesday, early in the morning, I received a call. I was told that the charge nurse was ill, there was no one who could take the charge nurse role and I was needed at work. My haircut would have to wait for a few more days. I made a call at six in the morning to the salon. I left a message telling them that I had been called into work unexpectedly and I would have to re-schedule my long overdue haircut. I also put the business card into my pocket, once again, and would try to remember to call and make sure the message was received. That day, again, I totally forgot to call the salon.

Once I go to work, my patients are my priority. When caring for critically ill patients, it is of utmost importance for the nurse not to be distracted. When I see nurses making calls to their mortgage broker to discuss escrow accounts, or restaurants to make reserva-tions for next week, or even surfing the Internet to find discount airline tickets, I wonder what is happening with their patients.

When I go to work, my mind must be at work; it cannot be with my hair specialist, it cannot be with my travel agent, and it cannot be anywhere except in that ICU with that patient. My mind, my entire attention, must be with my patients. My patients deserve all of me. I wouldn't want the nurse caring for my critically ill family member to be distracted by various reservations or appointments? I wouldn't want my family member to deteriorate while the nurse was surfing the Internet in search of anything other that the facts needed to provide them with the best care. I wouldn't want the nurse caring for my family to be distracted when her job is to provide quality care at all times? I know what I would want, and that is what I provide. That is why, every time I think I might have a few moments to make a personal phone call, I never accomplish that task.

When I go to work, my undivided attention is given to my patients. I give them the entire time for which I am being paid. I give them every moment of my day. And I give them quality care. That is what nurses should expect of themselves.

CHAPTER 19

At Peace with Death

My own personal experience with death. What can
you do for your own family member.

I have been asked, many times, how I deal with such a depressing job. The ICU is not always depressing; there are many times
when patients come to ICU, spend a few days, improve quickly,
and are transferred out of the unit to the medical floor. But there are
also many occasions when we must deal with death and dying. Because of the grave nature of the illnesses, the higher acuity of the
patients, and the unstable potentials, death is more common in the
ICU.

Death was not easy to deal with at first. As a young, inexperienced nurse, I would always fight to keep all my patients alive. Over
the years, I've learned that death is not always a bad thing. Sometimes death is best for the patient. I still work hard to save lives, but
once the health care team, the patient, and the family have established that there is no hope for survival, death may be a blessing.

It's easier to deal with deaths of those who are old, have lived a
long, fulfilled life, have no hope for a cure, or those who have suffered for an extended period of time. And it's also easier if the family members are supportive of the death. Those deaths are less stressful
because it seems to be the best for the patient. Often, the patients

know they are dying, but are hanging on for the family. Often, the patients are relieved when a family member gives them "permission" to die. Several times I have witnessed a family member say "it's OK to go," and the patient suddenly starts to deteriorate and quickly passes. It's these anticipated deaths that are easier, or even a sudden death of an older, terminally ill patient.

Whether it's expected or unexpected, old people or young, rich or poor, death is rarely an experience one looks forward to. There is always someone who is grieving and suffering. The ICU nurse becomes familiar with the signs of death and hopefully learns quickly how to make the passing of her patient a peaceful experience. Most of all, she must help to make this terrible experience as tolerable and pleasant as possible. The nurse who can support the patient and family through this experience will be remembered and appreciated forever.

* * *

I was called, one winter morning, and asked to support a family through the end-of-life experience with their loved one. This time, I was not the nurse caring for the patient, nor was I the charge nurse. I was the daughter-in-law. My husband received the call. His mother was in a hospital, halfway across the United States, and her condition was deteriorating. Mom had been taken to the hospital on Christmas Eve, suffering from a cold that had resulted in difficulty breathing. Because of her forty-year history of asthma, her lungs were in a weakened state, and at the age of eighty-eight, she was not going to survive this simple cold.

Upon arrival, Mom was admitted to the intensive care unit. Her oxygen level was dangerously low and her carbon dioxide level was excessively high. Her breathing was labored and, as expected, she was placed on bi-pap for ventilation support. The initial plan was to use this non-invasive support until Mom could "get over" her cold. But, after several days, it became more and more apparent that her simple cold resulted in a significant insult to her weakened lungs, and she may not be able to fight it off this time.

After four days she was still not improving. Usually, bi-pap is used for a day or two in order to help the patient get over the initial stage of a respiratory insult. In my experience, after a few days, the patient either improves, or intubation and initiation of a ventilator is needed. But, for Mom, neither alternative was an option. She was not getting better, and she was not going to be intubated. Mom had made her end-of-life wishes known to her husband, my father-in-law, many years ago. Mom was a retired nurse and well aware of her health risks and her options. She and Dad had completed all of the legal paperwork for a living will and each of them were aware of each other's desires.

On the fourth day, the doctors had the often-dreaded conversation with Dad about Mom's condition. Her prognosis looked poor; she was not responding to non-invasive treatment and a discussion about her end-of-life wishes was initiated. Dad discussed Mom's desires with her physician and as a result, as they finished the conversation, all agreed to initiate a "DNR" order. The medical team would continue to do whatever they could to help Mom survive this illness, but if something should happen and she would stop breathing or if her heart were to stop, the medical team would not intervene.

It was not necessary for Dad to ponder over this decision; he had been married to Mom for over sixty years and he knew, in his heart, what she would want. Many people go to the hospital, have DNR orders, and still regain their health enough to return home. Just because she had a DNR order did not mean she was definitely going to die. Dad remained close by Mom's side for the next twenty-four hours, but still no improvement. The next morning, the physician, once again, had a discussion with Dad about his wife's condition. It now was more apparent that she was not going to survive this illness. Each and every time the positive pressure mask was removed from Mom's face, either for face care, oral care, feeding, or to test her respiratory strength, her oxygen level plummeted. Now, five days into this illness, the doctors had to tell Dad that there was very little chance that his wife would survive. It was now time to take the next step and remove the positive pressure mask, which was keeping her alive, and let her die peacefully. That was when Dad initiated the phone calls to each of his children.

One son lived in the same town as his parents. He also had been visiting his mother on a daily basis and was continuing to hold out for hope of recovery. Two other sons came from the West Coast, and the only daughter came from the East Coast. And I, as the family nurse and the so-called expert, was summoned for my expertise and my experience with this type of situation. In all my years as a nurse, I have lived and experienced end-of-life situations more times than I can count. But this time it was different, this time I was on the other side. I would not be the nurse caring for the patient, I would not be the nurse explaining the events to the family, but I would be the family, I would be the grieving daughter-in-law. For the first time, I would be the one watching the nurse, or doctor, remove the life support from my loved one.

My father-in-law had requested, specifically, that I accompany my husband so I could "help with the situation." He wanted my opinion on everything that was happening. He needed me to confirm, what he already knew, that there were no other options available for our mom.

Within twenty-four hours of the phone calls, all of the children had arrived at the local airport. All four of them would be together, for the first time in over ten years, to support their father in the most difficult decision of his life.

As each of the children arrived, Dad made sure they read Mom's living will. Her wishes were spelled out very clearly. "No life support of any kind." And now was the time that her family had to abide by her wishes. In the early morning, I accompanied Dad to the hospital so we would be present when the doctors made their morning rounds. I spoke to each of her physicians about her condition. Was there a treatable illness? Was there any other option? What was the chance that she would recover? When the pulmonologist, the lung specialist, answered the last question with, "There is no chance for recovery," I knew we had no choice. I knew what we had to do.

At this time, my role moved into that grey area. I was no longer just the family member, yet neither was I the nurse in charge of this patient. I was now in a dual-role situation. I knew the nursing side, but I was technically on the other side. My nursing instincts kicked in. What I could do, and what I always do for my own patients, was to arrange for a family conference. This is a time when all the family members could sit in one room with the doctor, ask questions, receive answers, and hear the same information at the same time. Every family member must be in agreement with end-of-life decisions. Each one of them needs to be at peace with their own decision. Everyone must be on the same page in order for these traumatic situations to be successful.

Later that day, we had our conference. All the questions were answered. Everyone agreed that we had to do what Mom would want. We knew what we wanted, to keep her alive as long as possible, but we knew we had to do what Mom wanted. The time had come to do what she had asked, many years ago. The doctor wrote the orders to discontinue the positive pressure mask and provide comfort medication. He agreed that we could spend some time with her before removing the mask, and when we were ready, the nurse would assist us.

Mom was lethargic, tired, and exhausted from working hard just to breath. She had been using all of her energy for the past six days just to stay alive. She was still able to nod her head gently and squeeze our hands weakly upon request. After the family conference, Dad went to Mom's bedside. He spent some time with her, explaining that despite all of the medical efforts, her lungs were too weak to recover this time. He told her that he was going to abide by her wishes and remove the life support and allow her to go peacefully to God. The children gathered outside the room to allow Dad some time to tell Mom anything and everything he needed her to hear. After Dad was done, each one of us sat by Mom's bed, one-by-one, and reminded her once again that we loved her. Each of the children was allowed to say goodbye to the woman who had raised them and loved them for over fifty years.

After everyone had told her "I love you" and "goodbye," I once again had to change roles. I went to the nursing station and reported to the nurse that we were ready to remove the bi-pap. She assured me she would be there soon. I reminded her to bring the medication that would provide comfort as we prepared for a rapid ending. Within minutes, the nurse was at the bedside, performing the dreaded task that we had all agreed on. She removed the bi-pap mask, administered the medication, and asked if we needed anything else before she left the room to allow us to have our private time.

As we watched and waited, we continued to talk to Mom. She knew what was happening, she heard the conversations, and she was in agreement with all of the actions that were happening around her. She continued to breath fast and labored despite the comfort medication that was given. This was not what we wanted. We did not want her to continue to struggle for each breath. No one wanted her to suffer, which was why we were making the decision to allow for a peaceful death. Once I could see that the first dose of medication was not providing the relief Mom needed, I needed to switch roles again. I excused myself from the room and returned to the nursing station where I requested more medication. Now I was the nurse, once again. Now I needed to provide the comfort measures to the dying patient in the bed. The nurse reported that she would have to call the doctor for additional doses of medication. I agreed to wait patiently, but reminded her that we wanted a peaceful experience. "Tell the doctor, we want medication every thirty minutes," I asserted myself, knowing what I would request if I were in her shoes.

A few minutes later, the nurse was at the bedside with another injection. The doctor had not obliged my request for comfort medi-

cation every thirty minutes, but did provide an anti-anxiety medication for Mom—perhaps he should have provided six more doses,
one for each of us too. With this additional medication, Mom slipped
into a sleeping state. She could no longer respond to us, but we
were not certain that she didn't hear what we were saying. We all
remained at her bedside, reminiscing and telling stories that made
us all laugh and cry. We all supported each other as much as we
supported Mom during the last hours of her life.

During our family time at the bedside, I continued to play two
roles, the grieving family member, in my heart, and the nurse expert, in my mind. I answered the questions of the others, and tried
to reassure them that what we were experiencing was a natural, loving event.

"Can she hear us?" someone asked.

"Of course she can," I wanted them to talk as if she could hear
us. No one really knows when the dying stop hearing, but it is said
that it is the last of the senses to remain. As a nurse, I always assume
that my patient can hear everything that is said at the bedside. If
Mom could not hear what we were saying, it was still good to say it
out loud.

"What will happen if she doesn't have enough oxygen?"

Another question that I had to answer from my experiences as a
nurse, not as a family member. "As her oxygen level goes down, her
heart muscle will lose its ability to work, eventually her heart will
slow down and then stop."

"How low will her oxygen level go before her heart stops?"

That one I couldn't answer. "I don't know" There was no technical answer that I could provide for that question.

The nurses made sure we knew they were close. Each of them
asked permission to enter "our" room. Each of them continued to
provide personal care, turning, monitoring throughout the evening
as we held our vigil. Every nurse provided a professional presence
and supportive nature that was needed for our family. Initially, we
expected a quick passing, once the positive pressure mask was re-

moved. We expected her oxygen level to drop drastically and rap-idly, and a quick death to follow. But, we were wrong; someone else had a different plan. Mom remained with us for four hours after the positive pressure mask was removed. Mom was not in a hurry to leave her family who had gathered by her side for one last visit. She had what she loved, her family, and perhaps she was not so eager to leave that.

When the time came, and she was ready, her breathing pattern became more relaxed. We could see that it was now time for Mom to leave us, and move on to a wonderful place, a place where she could breath easy—something that she had not done for many years. We watched as her heartbeat slowly deteriorated and her breathing relaxed. We all stayed by her side as she slipped away.

I participated in this loving good-bye, as I have many times. But this time it was different. This time I didn't have to keep my distance to avoid showing my tear-filled eyes. This time I could stay at the bed-side and share tears with the family, because it was *my* family.

On that day, we gave Mom the best gift any one could give their family member. We allowed her to die with dignity. We didn't hold on because we loved her, but we let her go, because we loved her more. And she was at peace with her own death.

* * *

Death is a natural occurrence; we will all die some day. But none of us want to lose a loved one. We all want, for selfish reasons, to keep our family and friends alive as long as possible. No one wants to let go of Mom or Dad. We all want to keep them alive for ourselves. But, at the time of death, we cannot be selfish. We have to think of Mom or Dad and what is best for them, not what is best for us.

After seeing how many people deal differently with death, I now know there is no "right" way to handle it. Sometimes it's easier when the patient is older rather than younger. Sometimes it's easier when the patient has already suffered through a painful illness rather than a sudden event. But it is never easy.

What I have found is "right" is to allow the patient and the family to work through the dying process in whatever manner is most comfortable for them. If they want to discuss all options and make plans early, let them. If they don't want to talk about an impending death, don't pressure them. Allow the patient and the family to travel the path that they are most comfortable with. Be there to answer questions as they ask; be there to listen when they are ready to talk; and most of all, be there to support them as they determine their own needs.

I, personally, am an advocate of dying with dignity. When the time comes, it is best to allow a gentle passing rather than continue to try each and every medical intervention which may only slightly delay the inevitable. Sometimes the medical interventions will only prolong the suffering.

One of the best gifts a nurse can give to her patient is to support the patient and the family through a peaceful death. And, likewise, one of the best demonstrations of love a family member can give to their loved one is to allow a gentle and peaceful death.

We love you Mom, and that's why we let you go.

CHAPTER 20

Florence Nightingale in the ICU

The rewriting of the Florence Nightingale Pledge to meet the modernized world of nursing and especially in the ICU.

For many of us, Florence Nightingale is considered one of the "first" nurses. For many, she is the hero of nursing, and she has been credited with being the founder of modern nursing. Florence Nightingale, in my opinion, is the basis for what nursing is today. As I reviewed some of the published information on Florence Nightingale, I found the same information over and over in many references.

Nightingale was born in 1820, at a time when nursing was not viewed as a respectable profession. In the early days, nursing was not a profession for anyone of class. Nurses were seen as lower class individuals who were often thought of as promiscuous drunkards. During the lifetime of Florence Nightingale, she kept journal notes and wrote many books related to nursing. These writings have helped subsequent generations of nurses to understand where the profession was almost two-hundred years ago. When first entering the nursing profession, despite the objections of her family, Florence found conditions of over-crowding and filth that would hinder healing rather than promote healing. The sick were often sent to the hospital to die, perhaps because those who cared for them were uneducated and not adequately trained.

Some say Florence Nightingale was a modern woman before her times. She worked hard to change the conditions of the hospitals and the quality of nursing care. She did this, not because she was looking into the future, but because she was looking at the present and knew that what was not working in the 1800's, needed to be changed. She made those changes, and through her hard work, her speaking out, and her ongoing education of others, she helped to change nursing into a more respectable profession. It was during the era of Nightingale that the profession of nursing started to gain the respect it deserved. Today, we reap the benefits of her hard work and continue to promote nursing as a highly respectable profession.

Several of Nightingale's thoughts, follow along with my thoughts about the nursing profession. Many of those have already been shared throughout this book. One of her ideas was that she felt she "had a calling from God" to be a nurse and help others. I, too, believe that I had a calling. Maybe not in a spiritual manner, but I believe I was born to be a nurse. I wanted no other profession, at any time in my life. And I believe, as mentioned earlier in this book, that nurses are born, not trained, but maybe "called" to be nurses. Some people are meant to be nurses and some are not. Many, of whom I consider the best nurses, are those who have the same feelings that I do about a "calling" from an early age. Those who enter nursing for alternative reasons usually are not among the best of the nurses. Perhaps, the calling from a higher being, whatever or whomever we choose to believe, is the best explanation for the best nurses.

It was also written that Florence Nightingale believed that nursing was learned through experience, not through training. I, too, believe that experience is the best way to learn to be the best nurse. The newly graduated nurse has a lot to learn, just because they have learned theory in school, or practiced procedures in clinical rotations, doesn't mean they know everything they need to know. It takes experience to learn how to be a better nurse, how to deal with difficult situations, and to gain the intuition that makes the best nurses. I have learned this as I look back at some of my early nursing days and compare my actions to what I currently practice, after many years of experience.

Nightingale has also been quoted in one of her writings as saying we learn to think of our work, not ourselves. This is a reflection of how nurses strive to accommodate what is needed for their work and for their patients rather than what is needed for themselves. Many nurses work hard, they work long hours, and they do it for their patients. It is the caring nature of the nurse that makes her continue on, despite her own needs, and strive to assure all the needs of her patients are met.

Though Florence Nightingale was born almost 150 years before I was, we share several of the same thoughts and feelings of nursing. The calling that births the best nurses, the experience that makes the best nurses, and the fact that the best nurses will put the needs of their patients above their own.

When Florence Nightingale entered the hospital and found that overcrowding and filth was compromising the health of the patients, she started working toward making healthcare a better system. She was credited with reforming the hospital sanitation methods in order to prevent spread of infection and deaths. She worked hard to clean up the hospitals, prevent infections, provide quality care to her patients, and teach new nurses how to provide the same quality of care she felt was necessary. Patients needed the hospital to be a place where they could be helped, not harmed. Florence Nightingale was the foundation for what we know as nursing today. Her hard work and efforts laid the groundwork for promoting nursing as a highly skilled, respectable profession. A profession that many look up to today, no longer a profession of promiscuous drunkards, but respected professionals.

"Do no harm." Florence Nightingale suggested it many years ago, and today the entire medical profession is still based on that premise. Both the Hippocratic Oath for physicians and the Florence Nightingale Pledge for nurses promote the "Do no harm" premise.

＊ ＊ ＊

An oath is a pledge that one takes when promising to abide by rules that have been established by a specific group or organization. Doctors and nurses both have pledges that they abide by as they embark on their new careers. The physician's pledge, the Hippocratic Oath, reflects a code of medical ethics. It originated back in the 400's B.C. and was written by Hippocrates, who was considered by many as the "father of medicine." Hippocrates was a physician in Greece. When he started practicing medicine, many believed that illness was caused by superstitions, evil and disbelieving in God. He studied the human body, learned about diseases, and may have started one of the first medical schools based on his scientific reasoning.

Today, many graduating medical-school students swear to some form of the oath, usually a modernized version but the principles are the same, treat the sick to the best of one's ability, preserve patient privacy, teach the secrets of medicine to the next generation, and so on.

Hippocratic Oath—Classical Version

From *The Hippocratic Oath: Text, Translation, and Interpretation,*
by Ludwig Edelstein. Baltimore: Johns Hopkins Press, 1943.

I swear by Apollo Physician and Asclepius and Hygieia and Panaceia and all the gods and goddesses, making them my witnesses, that I will fulfill according to my ability and judgment this oath and this covenant:

To hold him who has taught me this art as equal to my parents and to live my life in partnership with him, and if he is in need of money to give him a share of mine, and to regard his offspring as equal to my brothers in male lineage and to teach them this art - if they desire to learn it - without fee and covenant; to give a share of precepts and oral instruction and all the other learning to my sons and to the sons of him who has instructed me and to pupils who have signed the covenant and have taken an oath according to the medical law, but no one else.

I will apply dietetic measures for the benefit of the sick according to my ability and judgment; I will keep them from harm and injustice.

I will neither give a deadly drug to anybody who asked for it, nor will I make a suggestion to this effect. Similarly I will not give to a woman an abortive remedy. In purity and holiness I will guard my life and my art.

I will not use the knife, not even on sufferers from stone, but will withdraw in favor of such men as are engaged in this work.

Whatever houses I may visit, I will come for the benefit of the sick, remaining free of all intentional injustice, of all mischief and in particular of sexual relations with both female and male persons, be they free or slaves.

What I may see or hear in the course of the treatment or even outside of the treatment in regard to the life of men, which on no account one must spread abroad, I will keep to myself, holding such things shameful to be spoken about.

If I fulfill this oath and do not violate it, may it be granted to me to enjoy life and art, being honored with fame among all men for all time to come; if I transgress it and swear falsely, may the opposite of all this be my lot.

This oath has been revised and rewritten several times in order to coincide with changes over time. The following is the updated version.

The Hippocratic Oath—Modernized Version

(Written by Louis Lasagna, Academic Dean of the
School of Medicine at Tufts University, 1964)

I swear to fulfill, to the best of my ability and judgment, this covenant:

I will respect the hard-won scientific gains of those physicians in whose steps I walk, and gladly share such knowledge as is mine with those who are to follow.

I will apply, for the benefit of the sick, all measures which are required, avoiding those twin traps of overtreatment and therapeutic nihilism.

I will remember that there is art to medicine as well as science, and that warmth, sympathy, and understanding may outweigh the surgeon's knife or the chemist's drug.

I will not be ashamed to say "I know not," nor will I fail to call in my colleagues when the skills of another are needed for a patient's recovery.

I will respect the privacy of my patients, for their problems are not disclosed to me that the world may know. Most especially must I tread with care in matters of life and death. If it is given me to save a life, all thanks. But it may also be within my power to take a life; this awesome responsibility must be faced with great humbleness and awareness of my own frailty. Above all, I must not play at God.

I will remember that I do not treat a fever chart, a cancerous growth, but a sick human being, whose illness may affect the person's family and economic stability. My responsibility includes these related problems, if I am to care adequately for the sick.

I will prevent disease whenever I can, for prevention is preferable to cure.

I will remember that I remain a member of society, with special obligations to all my fellow human beings, those sound of mind and body as well as the infirm.

If I do not violate this oath, may I enjoy life and art, respected while I live and remembered with affection thereafter. May I always act so as to preserve the finest traditions of my calling and may I long experience the joy of healing those who seek my help.

✳ ✳ ✳

Nurses also have a pledge, an adaptation of the physician's Hippocratic oath. It too, is considered to be the code of ethics for nursing. Lystra Gretter, a nursing instructor from Michigan, wrote this pledge in 1893. Unlike the Hippocratic oath, the nursing pledge was not written by the one who bears its name, but was named in honor of Florence Nightingale. The pledge, as originally written, is still often recited in pinning ceremonies and graduation ceremonies around the country.

The Florence Nightingale Pledge

(One and only version)

I solemnly pledge myself before God and in the presence of this assembly, to pass my life in purity and to practice my profession faithfully. I will abstain from whatever is deleterious and mischievous, and will not take or knowingly administer any harmful drug, I will do all in my power to maintain and elevate the standard of my profession, and will hold in confidence all personal matters committed to my keeping and all family affairs coming to my knowledge in the practice of my calling. With loyalty will I endeavor to aid the physician, in his work, and devote myself to the welfare of those committed to my care.

This pledge reflects the times in which it was written, 1893. Nurses in the nineteenth century were pledging to remain pure and faithful. This pledge, unlike the physician's Hippocratic Oath has never officially been revised or rewritten. Today nurses continue to recite this pledge at pinning and graduation ceremonies despite the outdated contents. The Hippocratic Oath has been revised several times to reflect the changing profession. The Nightingale Pledge, too, should be rewritten to reflect the changing nursing profession. In order to rewrite the pledge, first, let's look at what the pledge really means in the world of nursing today.

I solemnly—I take this oath seriously, not lightly, but with solid intensions of fulfilling a serious commitment to take good care of any and all sick people

pledge myself—I give you my word of honor because I am committed to provide the best care possible for all of my patients.

before God—Before any supreme being, my God or your God, to the doctors, to the administrators of the hospital, and especially to my patients, their families, and myself.

and in the presence of this assembly—In front of anyone and everyone, who will listen because I want everyone to know how strongly I feel about this and how proud I am to be a nurse.

to pass my life in purity—To live in a respectful manner that is reflective of the profession so highly respected by many. And to earn the respect that is deserved when I provide quality care.

and to practice my profession faithfully—To remain dedicated to those who will depend on me for all of their needs, and be trust worthy and reliable at all time.

I will abstain from whatever is deleterious and mischievous—I will maintain a safe environment for all those who are betrothed to my care.

And will not take—I will not take harmful substances that will impair my ability to perform and think intensively while on duty.

Or knowingly administer any harmful drug—I will not give any medications that may harm my patient.

I will do all in my power to maintain—I will continue learning on a daily basis because there are always opportunities to learn more innovative ways to provide quality care. And I will attend classes regularly to continue improving my skills and knowledge as long as I practice.

and elevate the standard of my profession—And provide nursing care according to current research because research based practice is most beneficial. I will teach other less experienced nurses who can learn from my experiences, and watch out for them when they try to do something dangerous, so they will someday provide even better care.

and will hold in confidence all personal matters committed to my keeping—I will maintain confidentiality at all times when in the best interest of my patients.

and all family affairs coming to my knowledge—And I will assure family is involved as much as possible because support from loved ones is more potent than any medication or treatments, especially for the dying patients.

in the practice of my calling—In any situation and opportunity

With loyalty—I will remain dedicated to the profession

will I endeavor to aid the physician, in his work—And help the physicians to provide the best care because I am with the patient many hours each day and he depends on me to relay pertinent information and act accordingly in order to provide urgent care.

and devote myself to the welfare of those—I will promote patient advocacy in order to assure the best care for all patients and I will remain devoted to my patients and provide them with my undivided attention while on duty.

committed to my care—as long as I practice nursing

* * *

After looking at the pledge and how it can be interpreted through modern eyes, and since it is no longer necessary that a nurse live her life in purity, I have chosen to rewrite the Florence Nightingale Pledge in a more modern version for all nurses.

The Florence Nightingale Pledge

(Revised for all nurses)

I give you my word of honor, to any supreme being, and to all here before me, to live in a respectful manner that is reflective of the profession, and remain dedicated, trustworthy and reliable. I will maintain a safe environment and avoid harmful substances that will impair my ability to provide quality care. I will not administer any medications that may be harmful. I will continue to expand my knowledge as long as I practice, and teach others who can learn from my experience. I will maintain confidentiality at all times and assure family is involved in the plan of care. With loyalty I will be respectful and help the physicians to do their work. I will remain devoted to my patients as long as I practice nursing.

✳ ✳ ✳

I have taken my experiences in the ICU to revise the Pledge even further. This time making it more specific to the ICU nurse, because the critical care area is a specialty area, with different kind of nursing.

The Florence Nightingale Pledge

(For the ICU Nurse)

I solemnly pledge to be the best ICU nurse I can be, and I promise to work endlessly on a daily basis. I will provide quality care to my critically ill patients who depend on me to live. I will abstain from harmful substances, because the smallest distraction could mean the difference between life and death. I will make sure all the physician orders are safe before performing them. I will not administer harmful drugs, but I will not consider harmful, those requested multiple doses of pain relievers and sedatives in order to reduce the suffering of a terminally ill patient.

I will do all in my power to maintain the highest knowledge base by continuing to seek learning experienced throughout my career. I will elevate the standard of the ICU nurse by sharing my knowledge with the less experienced. I will hold in confidence all personal matters as long as they don't interfere with my ability to properly care for my patient. I will encourage family involvement as much as possible for all patients, especially the dying. With loyalty and commitment, I will aid the physician, and the families in providing comfort to the seriously ill. I will promote advocacy in the best interest of all patients. And I will do my best to make sure every patient in my custody is provided with the best care possible at all times.

* * *

The Hippocratic Oath and the Florence Nightingale Pledge, state the obligation that physicians and nurses recite upon making the commitment to care for others. This commitment remains with them throughout their career life. These pledges, originated many years ago but still demonstrate the essence of the work. Both physicians and nurses are committed to maintaining the health of their patients. Both professionals never knowingly harm their patients, but strive daily to achieve the highest level of wellness for those who depend on them.

Whether reviewing the outdated Nightingale Pledge, or the updated version, everyone can see that nursing is a profession of dedicated, committed, educated, compassionate, helpers. Nurses must pledge to maintain high standards, and quality care for their patients. They must maintain a knowledge base and continuously strive to gain more knowledge and skills throughout their career, and they must pass those skills onto others of less experience. They pledge to provide the best care to the sick and ailing. The pledge demonstrates the dedication that nurses must have to provide what is expected in the helping profession they have chosen to pursue. Because of this dedication and perseverance, nursing has arrived at the level that would have made Florence Nightingale proud.

Who are You?

As you know by now, I have high standards for myself, for my fellow nurses, and for anyone who may be responsible to make medical decisions for another. There are many types of nurses and many types of people.

Are you?

… the nurse who takes the call bell away from the patient who calls too often?
or the nurse who puts the bell directly in the patient's hand for easy access?

… the person who refuses to consider that your young children may die from a traumatic accident?
or the person who talks to all your children and family members about donating organs, just in case of some traumatic accident?

… the nurse who puts diapers on the patient so she will not have to change the bed as often, despite the fact that the patient already has a diaper rash?
or the nurse who removes the diaper so she can see immediately when the patient is soiled and address the issue?

… the person who wants to keep your sick elderly parents alive on machines because you can't bear to be without them?
or the person who allows them to pass peacefully because death is easier than living on machines?

… the nurse who writes "poor appetite" because she doesn't want to make the time to feed her patient?

or the nurse who will help the patient feed himself bite by bite even if it means a shorter break?

… the person who develops impressions of others based on preconceived opinions?

or the person who gets to know every person before developing opinions?

… the nurse who focuses on tasks and writing everything down, rather than on the personal needs of the patient?

or the nurse who is so busy addressing all of the patients needs that she barely has time to document?

… the person who looses control and acts out in anger before you have all the facts?

or the person who stops and listens and learns before making any snap decisions and complaints?

… the nurse who gives her restless patient more medication to sedate him so she won't be bothered?

or the nurse who will sit by the bedside and talk and comfort him through his anxiety?

… the person who treats people differently based on who or what they are?

or the person who treats everyone the same, no matter who or what they are?

… the nurse who ignores the alarms because it's not her patient?

or the nurse who attends to all alarms because the safety of any patient is everyone's concern?

… the person who tries to avoid thinking about your parents or family members dying?

or the person who asks and talks about end-of-life decisions over and over again, so when the time comes, the decision will be easier?

… the nurse who turns her head when the patient who cannot talk is motioning for attention?

or the nurse who enters any room she walks by because the patient is motioning, even if it's not her patient?

Which nurse are you? Which nurse do you need to be?

Which person do you know you need to be?

Glossary

This is brief non-technical glossary for the non-professional reader. I have tried to explain, rather than define, any terms that have been used throughout the book. I hope readers find this helpful.

Medical Terms and Abbreviations

ABG's (Arterial Blood Gasses) – a test done with blood from the artery. The blood is most commonly drawn from the radial artery in the wrist. It is tested for oxygen, carbon dioxide, pH, and bicarbonate level. Expected results include a higher level of oxygen and a lower level of carbon dioxide. If the oxygen level is too low or the carbon dioxide level is too high it signifies that the patient is not adequately breathing. ABG's provide a direct measurement of oxygen saturation. Pulse oximeter measures an indirect oxygen saturation of the blood. (See O2 Sat).

Ambu Bag (Bag Valve Mask) – a hand held device that has a mask attached to a collapsible bag. This mask is placed on the victim's mouth and as the bag is squeezed, air is pushed into the lungs. Use of the ambu bag to ventilate a patient is frequently called "bagging" the patient.

Angioplasty – a procedure involving the inserting of a balloon into an obstructed blood vessel. The balloon is inflated, pressure is applied to the sides of the vessel, and the narrowed area is widened. Angioplasty is commonly done in the coronary arteries but can also be done in peripheral and renal arteries.

Arterial line (art-line) – a thin catheter inserted into an artery. It is usually inserted in the radial artery of the wrist, but sometimes in another location. The art-line allows minute-to-minute monitoring of blood pressure. It also provides access to draw ABG's and other lab specimens without repeatedly sticking the patient with a needles.

Bi-pap (Bi-level Positive Airway Pressure) – a form of non-invasive breathing support. It provides breathing support for patients without the invasion of an endotracheal tube. Bi-pap machines are similar to C-pap machines that some people use for sleep apnea. A facemask is positioned securely on the patients face. Tubing is attached from the facemask to the machine. The patient must have his/her own respiratory drive and be able to initiate breaths. Each time the patient initiates a breath the Bi-pap machine pushes oxygenated air into the lungs. This gentle pressure augments the shallow ineffective respirations. Bi-pap only assists ineffective breathing; it cannot breath for a patient.

Brain Death – the total irreversible loss of all brain activity. No brain function. There are no longer any thoughts, movements, or reflexes. When the brain is no longer functioning, the patient is dead. This is often difficult to understand because the patient may be on a ventilator that is pushing air into the lungs; the heart will continue to beat as long as it receives adequate oxygen. Most think if the heart is beating, the patient is alive. But in the case of brain death, this is not correct.

CABG (Coronary Artery Bypass Graft) – a surgery done to replace blocked coronary arteries. The new blood vessels are taken from various locations throughout the body, sometimes from the legs, from the arms, or from within the chest cavity. One end of the bypass graft is sewn onto the coronary artery distal to the blockage and the other end is attached to the aorta.

Cardiac Arrest – the sudden cessation of the heart. The heart stops beating, there is no pulse, and no blood circulating to the vital organs of the body. Immediate CPR must be started within 3-5 minutes to circulate the oxygenated blood and prevent brain damage.

Code Blue – the announcement that alerts the medical staff of a medical emergency usually indicating a patient requires immediate resuscitation, most often as a result of a cardiac arrest. Slang terms also used by medical professionals include: "code" by itself, as in "calling a code" or describing a patient as "coding".

Code Team – the group of staff members who respond to Code Blue calls. This team of experienced staff takes charge of emergency medical situations. Physician, nurse, orderlies, respiratory therapist, nursing supervisor, EKG technician, and pharmacist may make up the Code Team. Each hospital may call it something different and have a different combination of people, but the goal is the same.

CPR (Cardio-Pulmonary Resuscitation) – the combination of artificial blood circulation with chest compression and artificial respirations with mouth-to-mouth ventilation. CPR is not likely to restart the heart, but rather its purpose is to maintain a flow of oxygenated blood to the brain thereby delaying brain damage.

Crash Cart – the mobile cart that is rolled to Code Blue events. The cart is stocked with a variety of equipment needed in emergency situations.

Crashing – a slang term nurses use to alert others that the patient's condition is deteriorating. When one nurse says to another, "My patient is crashing." the second nurse is immediately aware of a crucial situation.

CRRT (Continuous Renal Replacement Therapy) – a form of dialysis. Unlike dialysis—performed for a few hours each day—CRRT is done continuously throughout the 24-hour period. CRRT is a slower filtration of the blood and is used for unstable patients who cannot tolerate the rapid removal of fluids through the traditional dialysis therapy.

CVP line (Central Venous Pressure line) – a thin catheters inserted in a large central vein. Usually inserted in the neck or upper chest. CVP lines allow for administration of large volumes of fluids, monitoring CVP pressure or fluid balance, and the administration of medications that are irritating to peripheral veins.

Defibrillate – a term for the delivery of a small dose of electrical energy to the heart. "Shocking" the cardiac muscle may terminate the irregular rhythm and allow the heart to return to the normal rhythm. External defibrillators, with paddles, are used in cardiac arrest.

AED's (Automatic External Defibrillators) are seen more and more in public places and allow lay people the ability to intervene rapidly in the event of a cardiac arrest.

Internal defibrillators are inserted along with pacemakers for patients who have had previous cardiac arrests and/or lethal irregular heart rhythms.

Dialysis – replaces the function of the kidneys—is the treatment of renal failure. A special access device, like a large IV catheter, is inserted and the patient is connected to a dialysis machine for a few hours at a time. As the patient's blood flows through the machine, the toxins are filtered. Patients with chronic renal failure will go to dialysis centers for a few hours three times each week. More acutely ill patients may require dialysis daily or every other day.

DNR (Do-Not-Resuscitate) – a directive that alerts the medical professionals that resuscitation should not be attempted if a person suffers a cardiac or respiratory arrest. Any person who does not wish to undergo life sustaining treatment can request a DNR order. DNR is more commonly done when a patient is suffering from an irreversible illness, is deemed terminally ill, and desires a more natural death. To the healthcare providers, this means if the heart stops or the patient stops breathing, the nurses will provide comfort care and allow for a more natural and peaceful death.

Drips – the slang used by nurses and doctors to indicate that a patient is on a continuous IV infusion of medications. Drips most often refer to the medications that are adjusted by the nurse, based on parameters to keep blood pressure, heart rates, and sedation levels in a predetermined range.

DT's (delirium tremens) also called alcohol withdrawals. The episode of anxiety, confusion, and/or hallucinations along with shakiness and uncontrolled tremors that occur after a long period of drinking is stopped abruptly. They usually start a few days after alcohol consumption is stopped and lasts about three to ten days, but varies depending on the severity of the problem. DT's can cause seizures and even death if not prevented and/or treated carefully.

End-of-life wishes – the term used to describe medical care options for patients who are considered irreversibly ill. This may be a patient with a terminal illness like cancer or a patient who has a sudden illness deemed incurable. End-of-life care includes comfort measures, pain medication, personal care support, and especially emotional support for both the patient and the family.

Endotracheal Tube (ET tube, ETT) – a tube that is inserted, through the mouth or the nose, into the trachea. After the tube is placed in the airway it can be attached to an ambu-bag or a ventilator. The process of inserting an ETT is called intubation.

Intubate/Intubation—the process of inserting an ET tube.

Intravenous (IV) catheter – a small plastic catheter that is inserted into the vein. The IV allows for infusion of fluids and medications directly into the blood stream.

Intra-aortic balloon pump (IAPB) – A cardiac assist machine. A ballooned catheter is inserted through the femoral artery and threaded up toward the heart. The balloon lays in the aorta. It inflates and deflates with each heartbeat. The synchronous inflation and deflation of the balloon helps to increase blood flow to the coronary arteries and takes the workload off the heart.

Life-Support – any treatment, medications, interventions and therapies that prolong the patient's life when essential body systems are not functioning sufficiently to sustain life unaided. Any treatment that if removed, would result in the patient's death. Some life support therapies include: mechanical ventilation with a ventilator, Bi-pap if the patient can't breath sufficiently without it, medications supporting the blood pressure, feeding tubes providing nourishment, pacemakers, and dialysis.

Monitor – the machine at the bedside that displays various waveforms and numbers. The display includes EKG rhythm, heart rate, blood pressure, respiratory rate, and oxygen saturation for most patients. In addition, waveforms from Art lines, CVP lines, PA lines, and intracranial pressure monitoring can be displayed on the monitor.

Mouth-To-Mouth ventilation involves one person making a seal between their mouth and the patient's mouth and 'blowing', in order to push air into the patient's lungs. It is a vital part of CPR, mostly used by the lay rescuer. Medical personnel have ambu-bags or other types of equipment to use instead of their mouth.

Organ Donation – the removal of vital organs—heart, lungs, liver, kidneys, pancreas and more— after the patient has recently died. Organs are removed from a brain dead patient for the purpose of transplanting.

O2 Sat (Oxygen Saturation) – the number measured by the pulse oximeter. O2 Sat is measured with a sensor that looks like a white band-aid and is most often placed on a finger. This band-aid is attached to a wire that leads to the bedside monitor. A red light shines from the band-aid device, through the finger, toe, or earlobe that it is attached to, and reads the amount of oxygen circulating in the red blood cells of the body. This provides an indirect measurement of the patients oxygen level at all times.

PRN – an acronym for the Latin phrase *pro re nata*, which means "for the thing born". In medicine PRN means, "as needed." It is used for medications, treatments and other interventions that can be initiated on-and-off rather than regularly scheduled. Examples include: medicate prn pain, breathing treatments prn wheezing.

Pulmonary Artery Lines (PA line) – a catheter inserted through a large vein and threaded through the right side of the heart into the pulmonary artery of the lungs. This important catheter allows for direct measurement of pressures from the heart and lungs. It allows the medical team to monitor fluid balance and the function of the heart.

Rapid Response Team – a medical emergency team that brings critical care expertise to the bedside. This team is activated for urgent situations when a nurse needs assistance with a clinical situation that requires a higher level of support. Various facilities include different people in their teams, but most often include a critical care nurse and a respiratory therapist.

Respiratory Arrest – the cessation of breathing. It is a medical emergency that requires mouth-to-mouth ventilation or intubation, and will be followed with ventilator support. If untreated, will be followed by cardiac arrest.

Respiratory Therapist (RT) – a health professional that specializes in the assessment and treatment of respiratory pathologies. They are specialists in airway management and mechanical (artificial) ventilation. They provide vital support to the medical team and work closely with nurses and doctors in the critical care area.

Restraints are soft fabric ties used to constrict movement. Medical restraints are used as a last resort to prevent patients from harming themselves or others. Lap belts may be used to prevent patients from falling. Limb restraints can be used to prevent patients from pulling at life-support tubes.

Saline Lock – a short tubing attached to the IV catheter. The tubing is flushed with normal saline and clamped. No IV solution runs through the saline lock. It remains in place to allow for quick IV access in case the patient needs emergency medications.

Telemetry – usually refers to wireless communication. In the hospital setting it is used for patients who require EKG monitoring. EKG electrodes are attached to the patient's chest and connected to a transmitting device. Patients can walk around with the portable transmitter (tele box) while their heart rhythm is monitored remotely.

Tissue Donation – the removal of tissues such as corneas, bones, skin, heart valves, and veins that can be taken from patients after death and used for other living persons in need. Corneas can be transplanted to allow a blind person to see, skin and bone can be used for grafts, heart valves and veins can be used for various surgeries. In some states—like California—laws mandate that ALL deaths be reported to the donor network. The network staff will review each patient for potential donation and contact family if indicated.

Tracheostomy (Trach) – the surgical procedure physicians perform to place the breathing tube, through a hole in the neck, directly into the trachea. This usually replaces the ET tube after it is determined the patient will need long term ventilation support. The surgeon makes a small incision between the collarbones and inserts a shortened tube directly into the airway. This tube is then attached to the ventilator and the ET tube can be removed from the mouth.

Vasopressors – substances that cause vasoconstriction—the narrowing of blood vessels. Patients who are in shock or suffering from a critical illnessess may have life threatening low blood pressure. Generalized vasoconstriction will increase the systemic blood pressure and increase blood circulation to vital organs. Vasopressor "drips" are infused and adjusted according to prescribed parameters.

Ventilator – a machine designed to mechanically move air into and out of the lungs. The ventilator is attached to the endotrachael tube or the tracheostomy tube. It is used when the patient is physically unable to breathe, or breathing inadequately.

Diseases

Amyotrophic Lateral Sclerosis (ALS) also known as Lou Gehrig's disease is a degenerative neurological disease caused by a degeneration of the nerve cells in the spinal cord that controls voluntary muscle movement. The disorder causes muscle weakness throughout the body when the nerves cease to send messages to the muscles. The cognitive function is usually spared leaving the mind totally intact, but the body useless.

Alcoholism is a disease caused by the addiction to alcohol. Alcoholism results in the daily consumption of alcoholic beverages despite negative consequences.

Aneurysm is a localized dilation of a blood vessel. The balloon-like bulge is caused by a weakening of the vessel wall. Aneurysms are most commonly found in the arteries of the brain and the aorta. As the size of an aneurysm increases, the wall weakens, and the risk of rupture is more likely. A ruptured aneurysm can result in severe hemorrhage and sudden death.

Asthma is a chronic lung disease characterized by inflammation and obstruction of the upper airways. Asthma "attacks" can be treated with medications.

Bipolar Disorder (also known as Manic-Depressive Disorder) is a psychiatric diagnosis characterized by mood disorders. Individuals experience manic episodes of abnormally elevated moods, periods of depressive episodes of abnormally low moods, and sometimes mixed episodes where both mania and depression are present at the same time. Abnormal moods are separated by periods of normal moods.

Chronic Obstructive Pulmonary Disease (COPD) is a chronic disease of the lungs resulting in narrowed airways and shortness of breath. Unlike asthma COPD is rarely reversible and usually gets progressively worse over time. Long history of smoking can cause COPD.

Diabetes (Diabetes Mellitus) is a metabolic disorder resulting from abnormally high blood sugar levels. Diabetes is usually cause by heredity and environmental causes. Obesity is a common precursor to diabetes.

Guillain-Barré is an autoimmune disease that affects the peripheral nervous system. It is usually triggered by an infection or virus. Minor generalized weakness followed by more significant weakness, and finally, if untreated, total paralysis. The paralysis usually starts with the lower extremities and progresses upward to include the arms and the chest.

Incision and Drainage (I & D) is usually a minor surgical procedure—a small incision or puncture—to release a build up of pus from an abscess, boil or encapsulated infection. By opening the skin, the infected drainage can escape and the abscess will heal.

Intracranial Hemorrhage (ICH) is bleeding within the skull. Blood accumulates in the brain tissues as a result of trauma, fall, motor vehicle accident, etc. Because the skull is bone and cannot expand, the pressure of the blood in the brain presses on the brain tissue and causes neurological changes. Strokes can be caused by ICH.

Myocardial Infarction (MI) commonly called a heart attack occurs when the oxygenated blood supply to the heart muscle is blocked. Usually due to a blocked coronary artery that restricts blood flow from reaching any area of the heart muscle. If untreated that area of the heart muscle that is starved of blood will die. Unlike other muscles of the body, the cardiac muscle does not regenerate and heal—once dead, always dead.

Morbidly Obese – According to the United States National Institutes of Health (NIH), the term "morbid obesity" is defined as being 50-100 percent above one's ideal body weight, or 100 pounds above one's ideal body weight. A person with a BMI (body mass index) value of 40 or greater would also be considered morbidly obese. Medical problems commonly resulting form morbid obesity include diabetes, high blood pressure, heart disease, stroke, sleep apnea, heart failure and ultametly death.

Multiple Sclerosis (MS) is a chronic autoimmune condition in which the immune system attacks the nervous system of the body. MS affects the ability of nerve cells in the brain and spinal cord to communicate with each other. It is a progressive disease that results in a larger variety of manifestations including muscle weakness, paralysis, and can result in mental deterioration towards the end of the illness.

Obesity is a condition in which excessive body fat has negatively affected the health of the person. Obesity is defined as a body mass index (BMI) of more than 30. Obesity in America is rising rapidly and quickly becoming an epidemic resulting in multiple health problems.

Pancreatitis is the inflammation of the pancreas. Often cause by gallstones, excessive alcohol intake, and a variety of less common reasons.

Schizophrenia is a psychological disorder that may be characterized by abnormal thoughts of reality. Commonly manifested by paranoia, delusions, disorganized speech and thoughts.

Sepsis is a medical condition characterized by a whole-body inflammation as a result of an infection. The infection usually starts in another organ, bladder, lungs, abscess and spreads to the blood. The inflammation causes a shock state called "septic shock" resulting in low blood pressure, respiratory distress, organ failure, and will cause death if untreated.

Subarachnoid Bleed is blood in the area surrounding the brain. It may occur spontaneously, from a ruptured aneurysm, or from trauma of head injury.

Reference, see www.wikipedia.org

LaVergne, TN USA
23 February 2010
174009LV00009B/40/P